Person-centred Health Care

T0258571

Person-centred health care is increasingly endorsed as a key element of high-quality care, yet, in practice, it often means patient-centred health care. This book scrutinizes the principle of primacy of patient welfare, which, although deeply embedded in health professionalism, is long overdue for critical analysis and debate. It appears incontestable because patients have greater immediate health needs than clinicians and the patient–clinician encounter is often recognized as a moral enterprise as well as a service contract. However, Buetow argues that the implication that clinician welfare is secondary can harm clinicians, patients and health system performance.

Revaluing participants in health care as moral equals, this book advocates an ethic of virtue to respect the clinician as a whole person whose self-care and care from patients can benefit both parties, because their moral interests intertwine and warrant equal consideration. It then considers how to move from values including moral equality in health care to practice for people in their particular situations. Developing a genuinely inclusive concept of person-centred care – accepting clinicians as moral equals – it also facilitates the coalescence of patient-centred care and evidence-based health care.

This reflective and provocative work develops a constructive alternative to the taken-for-granted principle of primacy of patient welfare. It is of interest to students and academics in the health and caring sciences, philosophy, ethics, medical humanities and health management.

Stephen Buetow is Associate Professor of General Practice and Primary Health Care at the University of Auckland, New Zealand. He is also an Honorary Professor at Queen Margaret University in Edinburgh, Scotland, and Associate Editor of the *Journal of Evaluation in Clinical Practice* and the *European Journal for Person Centered Healthcare*.

Routledge Advances in the Medical Humanities

Person-centred Health Care

Balancing the welfare of clinicians and patients

Stephen Buetow

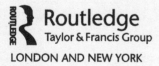

Routledge
Taylor & Francis Group

LONDON AND NEW YORK

First published 2016 by Routledge

2 Park Square, Milton Park, Abingdon, Oxfordshire OX14 4RN

52 Vanderbilt Avenue, New York, NY 10017

Routledge is an imprint of the Taylor & Francis Group, an informa business

First issued in paperback 2019

British Library Cataloguing-in-Publication Data
A catalogue record for this book is available from the British Library

Library of Congress Cataloging-in-Publication Data
Names: Buetow, Stephen, author.
Title: Person-centred health care : balancing the welfare of clinicians and
patients / Stephen Buetow.
Other titles: Routledge advances in the medical humanities.
Description: Abingdon, Oxon ; New York, NY : Routledge, 2016. | Series:
Routledge advances in the medical humanities | Includes bibliographical
references and index.
Identifiers: LCCN 2015050381| ISBN 9781138819771 (hardback) |
ISBN 9781315744247 (ebook)
Subjects: | MESH: Primary Health Care | Physician-Patient Relations
Classification: LCC R727.3 | NLM W 84.61 | DDC 610.69/6–dc23
LC record available at http://lccn.loc.gov/2015050381

ISBN: 978-1-138-81977-1 (hbk)
ISBN: 978-0-367-28071-0 (pbk)

Typeset in Galliard
by Wearset Ltd, Boldon, Tyne and Wear

For my late father, John Buetow, and my mother, Diane Buetow (née Schneideman).

Contents

Acknowledgements

This book could never have been written without direct support from others. Most important has been Esther – my wife and best friend – who has stood by me, providing love and understanding, emboldening me to continue writing the book when I have doubted myself. Esther read and provided feedback on the whole book, which is cause in itself for my appreciation.

My publisher, Routledge (Taylor & Francis), has encouraged and supported me from the start of this venture, in particular via editorial assistance from Louisa Vahtrick and Fergus Paton. The Staffing Committee of the Faculty of Medical and Health Sciences at the University of Auckland approved and funded the Research and Study Leave that permitted me to work full-time on the book during the 2015 calendar year. My school and department at the university accommodated this period of absence. Harvard Art Museums provided me with the image shown as Figure 2.1 and authorized me to use it in this book.

My leave allowed me to travel overseas to conduct research for the book. Hosting my visits were: the Gothenburg Centre for Person-Centred Care, King's College London, London South Bank University, Oxford University, Edinburgh's Queen Margaret University, Stony Brook University and the University of Toronto. I also benefitted from involvement with the European Society for Person-Centered Health Care, especially Andrew Miles, and its June 2015 conference at Madrid's Francisco de Vitoria University. Beyond these targeted visits, I received advice or feedback on individual chapters, sections of chapters, or particular issues from academic and professional colleagues: Yvonne Bray, Susan Carter, Bruce Charlton, Karen Day, Thomas Fröhlich, Natalie Gauld, Rabbi Mendel Goldstein, Marcus Henning, Peter Huggard, Tim Kenealy, John Kennelly, Lani Lopez, Michael Loughlin, Rod McLeod, Brendan McCormack, Ruth Spence, Joachim Sturmberg and Craig Webster. However, I take full responsibility for all errors of omission and commission in this book.

1 Introduction

I had become my swollen testicle. To the junior physician in one of Australasia's busiest Emergency Departments, it defined me as an object of clinical investigation. Differentiating me from the other men in my ward – caged in the same bleached, anonymizing gowns – it centred his care in a reductionist and mechanical culture of standardized proceduralism. The implications of this cool semblance of professionalism disconcerted me. Categorizing me by my complaint excised the need of the physician to care for me as unique and complex, as a person who might not fit standard operating guidelines for conveyor belt medicine. In so acting, the physician reduced himself to an embodied social function, losing the opportunity to partner with me to optimize our interrelated experience for mutual care.

To assert my personhood, I recounted the background to my presenting condition. Despite no sound privacy in my cubicle, I told the physician what I had just told several nurses: that I had experienced similar symptoms of testicular pain and swelling of sudden onset multiple times in previous decades. They had first presented in my twenties. Invariably they abated within 24 hours – typically, straight after an ultrasound scan ruled out testicular torsion. I had hoped my physician would apply William Osler's directive to 'Listen to your patient, he is telling you the diagnosis.' By trusting my coherent narrative, he could have relied less on common, pre-established diagnostic categories; not quizzed me about my sex life; and not insisted on collecting urine and blood samples to rule out an infection. He would have recognized my history of partial torsion and its recurring expression through the co-emergence of storied states of my body, mind and lived experience. Managing my medical condition as a potential emergency, he would have expedited the scan I requested, while showing empathy for my 'dis-ease'.

When the scan I eventually received revealed no pathology, I was returned as a low-acuity patient to my ward for further protracted waiting without information on the next step in my care. Feeling abandoned and that I was wasting everyone's time, I discharged myself 'against medical advice'. Within the hour my symptoms resolved, validating in my mind my decision to go home early.

Reports like mine – of patients feeling dehumanized and a burden – are ubiquitous in health care. They illustrate unmet needs for health systems to improve the experience of patients – who lack the power and other resources of clinicians – by overtly respecting them as *persons*. Patient-centred health care has been revitalized to help meet this need in the light of population health goals.

However, concern for patients' perspectives and experience is insufficient. As my story shows, it provides only a partial account that tends to neglect how the personhood of the clinician is morally important for itself and its impact on patient welfare. My physician cannot speak here for himself but I have imagined how the circumstances in which he attended me might have shaped his experience and, indirectly, mine. The emergency department was a high stress environment in which demonstrating respect and concern for personhood challenged everyone, including him. His high workload was visible. He was a busy young man working a late night shift in an overcrowded hospital. Many of his acutely unwell patients were distressed and some were audibly challenging. Unable to access my medical records to verify my story, he was disadvantaged by not knowing me and by difficulties in getting to know his patients as persons. Presumably his clinical supervisor expected him to follow and document a task-oriented clinical checklist. This standardizing of care compromised his developing clinical skills and freedom to manage complex variation. On top of all this, no urology registrar or consultant was readily available to support my inexperienced physician so late at night.

For all these reasons I sensed his vulnerability and own need for care in the complex system in which we had been thrown together. Improving his capacity and mine to co-produce care for our interconnected welfare required us to recognize and manage our interdependence to shared advantage. Put simply, my welfare and his were mutually reinforcing. The moral synergisms between our respective interests highlighted a bounded but unmet need and opportunity for reciprocated care – care exchanged between the clinician and patient to enable us each to flourish as persons in just and caring terms. The widely used model of *patient-centred* health care is ill-equipped to manage this opportunity.

Patient-centred health care recognizes the importance of the health of the patient as a person but lacks sufficient focus on how the welfare of the clinician impacts the care of the patient. Any acknowledgement by this model that the clinician, no less than the patient, is a person too is almost parenthetical. Without attending to moral values and personal virtues, the model focuses on the professional duty of the clinician to produce, with the patient, care directly *for the patient* even though the welfare of each party is positively interrelated. This inequality in care struggles to be functional for patient welfare because it weakens clinicians, who commonly neglect themselves and experience unwellness, while population health goals can also undermine patients' personal care. Yet, these limitations of patient-centred care create the moral space to implement *person-centred* health care.

Rather than take the spotlight off care of the patient, person-centred health care enlarges this light to illuminate the patient and clinician as persons beyond these particular social roles. Person-centred health care seeks to maximize the welfare of persons who – by nature of being persons – have fundamentally equal moral worth within a professional relationship of interdependency. More concretely, the greater inherent dependency of the patient than the clinician within this relationship necessitates patients gaining directly from clinician care and patient self-care, but also indirectly when clinician welfare is protected within health care teams including clinicians and patients.

Evolutionary rather than revolutionary therefore, person-centred health care aims to build on the care of the patient as a person by balancing and bridging the moral interests of each party. To co-produce 'win–win' care for moral reasons faithful to the personhood of the patient and clinician, it uses dialogue and, if necessary, deliberation informed by developing and expressing good character. Deeply rooted values nourish inculcated virtues that dispose the patient and clinician to live well and blossom.

I wish to introduce these issues more fully now to undergird my overview of the structure and style of this book on what is needed to move from the ideal of patient-centred health care toward person-centred health care. In my Emergency Department story, a person-centred physician would have gone beyond efficiently managing the scan that I had come to expect over two decades of presenting with the same medical problem. The scan was clinically necessary for my welfare, socially just and requested by me. Giving it without fuss would have made my care patient-centred. It would have put my welfare first – but it would not have *maximized* my welfare or that of my *physician*. Real victory for us both, requiring little time or effort on his part, would have set in motion an end to my repeated emergency visits. Recognizing that my medical history made likely another negative scan, my physician could have gently garnered before this test my ready commitment to access follow-up medical care if the scan revealed no disease. That future care could prevent my symptoms recurring and fix, at last, my increased risk of complete torsion. Person-centred health care would also have helped me to acquire and exercise good character for joint benefit, a theme I will return to later.

Moral crisis

My story adds to mounting evidence of a moral meltdown in health care – 'a crisis of knowledge, compassion, care and costs'.[1] More insidious than the health care scandals and total failures that periodically stun all health systems, this moral crisis – or at least an urgent need to recalibrate moral practice in modern health systems – reflects a pervasive cultural malaise: the 'depersonalization' of patients and clinicians, in its de-humanizing and de-individuating senses. Since the development of modernity and the bureaucratic state, this depersonalization has been growing, most recently with empirical science steadily appropriating social life – not only health care. As a consequence, it is especially disconcerting that in the name of care, much health care appears uncaring.

Caring signifies what matters to people. Despite – if not because of – the growth in advances in science and new and emerging information and communication technologies, patients and clinicians are struggling to interrelate as moral agents who care for themselves and each other. I do not wish to diminish celebrating scientific advances and their contribution to gains in human health and welfare. However, these gains have come at a high social cost. Health care has become increasingly based on, rather than merely informed by, scientific developments. Scientism threatens personal identity and intimacy, trumping calls for an open, more caring society[2,3] to replace one that – more and more – devalues and marginalizes caring as a duty within social spaces of blurred sincerity and insincerity. In the midst of this Cassandra phenomenon, health systems require clinicians to put patients first.

Yet neither patients nor clinicians are commonly treated as people – as ends within interdependent relations – by these fragmented, standardized and anonymizing systems. In these systems for health and welfare, strangers care increasingly for strangers. The personhood of patients and clinicians becomes imperceptible as systems lose their ability to discern it. Personhood is lost from the human need of patients and clinicians – as people who share vulnerability to disease and death – to feel interconnected, understood and valued equally for their equal moral worth and dignity. Illustrating how a sense of personhood has become obscured is a proposal, recently published in the *Journal of the American Medical Association*, to consider banning handshakes from clinical care in order to limit the spread of infection.[4] Their proposal extends American physician Lewis Thomas'[5] concern that 'Medicine is no longer the laying on of hands. It is more like the reading of signals from machines'. For example, intensive care unit procedures – none of which involves touch – have been equated mnemonically with giving a 'Fast hug'.[6] If only understanding were increased – for example from Raymond Carver's poem, *What the Doctor Said* – of how touch can enable clinicians and patients to learn and bridge their symbolic spaces through healing communion. It is no wonder that health systems struggle to enable and motivate clinicians, from a sense of moral vocation, to care for themselves and patients who trust them. Exacerbating this supply issue is the rising demand for health care.

This demand from clinicians, patients and others is taking place as patients, within ageing populations, are living longer with chronic health conditions, multi-morbidity, disability and frailty. Patients are looking beyond cure, which is not always achievable, for compassion and comfort through personal health care delivery that normatively combines intimacy with an appropriate degree of social distance. Progress toward these ends is slowly taking place. Costly modern health systems are beginning to move away from an impersonal, one-size-fits-all model of fix-it, industrialized patient care. However, personalization is acquiring a narrow meaning that is unsatisfying in its incompleteness.

Advancing biotechnologies in areas like molecular medicine, genomics and bioinformatics are personalizing medical care. These technologies enable prevention and treatment programmes to manage individual patient risks rather than group risks. Personalized risk information promises to empower patients to increase control over their health care. However, this promise is empty unless the information predicts health risks that patients can act on to reduce disease and mortality. Moreover, personalized medicine is silent on addressing social determinants of population health like poverty, and relational caring of patients as people – which cannot be 'tacked on to biomedicine'.[7] Faithful to another of Osler's maxims, 'It is much more important to know what sort of patient has a disease than what sort of disease a patient has', such caring has been suggested to require integrating 'personomics' into precision medicine.[8] Yet, clinician welfare is also still marginalized even though clinicians are people too and need their welfare revalued as 'less a private matter ... [than] something closer to a shared resource'.[9] Thus, unmet needs remain to enable patients and clinicians to experience caring, balance their welfare and flourish – needs eclipsing the scope of evidence for patient care.

Consideration is required of the shared need of clinicians and patients to care, and be cared for, beyond burgeoning developments in science. Evidence-based medicine epitomizes the difficulty of accounting for humanistic interests of both parties. This model struggles to explain cogently how to reconcile patients' and clinicians' values and sources of knowledge when these different inputs conflict, and move with prudent compassion from evidence to personalized moral action. Each time that this model reconstitutes itself to try to address these concerns it becomes less faithful to its misleading name. This book therefore responds not merely to an epistemological transition of what counts as knowledge but also to a fundamental, axiological widening of awareness of what people care about within health care. Adding to my concern to revive – before cure – the importance of caring, compassion, comfort and consolation is the unhelpful reassertion by health systems of their commitment to patient-centredness.

Patient-centred health care

In the roles of critic and conscience, patient-centred health care has proven ineffective in holding evidence-based medicine to account – perhaps because, in common with consumerism, evidence-based medicine checks a powerful medical profession. However, contemporary primary care reforms in the United States have promoted patient-centred, population health care models, like the patient-centred medical home, to improve quality in health care and reduce costs. Developments of this type have revised and revived the importance of patient-centred health care such that a leading general medical journal in the United States recently opened its editorial by blandly asserting, as a mere truism, that, 'Nearly every medical student and practicing physician aspires to provide the best possible patient-centered care.'[10] Nursing tends to make the same kind of assumption whose apparent self-evidence acts against critical scrutiny amid widespread confusion around what patient-centred health care actually entails;[11] for the meaning of patient-centred health care 'is at once obvious and obscure'.[11]

What is clear is that patient-centred health care stipulates the duty of the clinician to put first the welfare of the patient. This care aspires to be *for* each patient as the only patient in a manner that also emanates *from* the patient's full involvement in health care. Patients have greater immediate health care needs than the clinician, and the knowledge, experiences and preferences of patients can guide clinicians to help manage these needs. My appreciating these commitments however does not negate my viewing them with suspicion. Patients are not always sick, and people, including clinicians, can be unwell without adopting the role of patient. Thus, for example, ought the welfare of tired and depressed clinicians, who refuse health care, necessarily be distinguished from, and come second to, the welfare of all the patients they treat? By answering 'yes', patient-centred health care effectively encourages clinicians to neglect their own welfare, which compromises their ability to care for patients.

To fix the false economy of not looking after clinicians, health systems have made progress in attending to clinician health and sustainable practice. However, failure to address the underlying issue of clinicians' sacrifices for patients' welfare has contributed to widespread clinician unwellness. Positively related to perceived errors in health care,[12] work-related stress and burnout among clinicians continue to threaten the safety and effectiveness of health care teams and patient care. What is bad for clinicians is seldom good for patients; yet despite recognizing the patient as a person, patient-centred health care speaks in an undertone to the clinician-as-person, harming clinicians and patients.

This relative lack of care for clinicians and other carers indicates that one-sided benefits to patients are pyrrhic for clinicians. In turn, welfare gains are subprime for patients because, like Sisyphus, they ascend toward but never reach the pinnacle of full interdependence and mutual flourishing. As Charles Bardes explained in the *New England Journal of Medicine*,[13] 'The flaw in the metaphor [of patient-centredness] is that the patient and the doctor must coexist in a therapeutic, social and economic relation of mutual and highly interwoven prerogatives'. However, Bardes added that 'Neither is the king, and neither is the sun', whereas I contend that each is the king and each is the sun, and thus that patient-centred health care errs in casting the clinician as the shadow on the patient sun. The clinician–patient relationship should be not patient-centred but a purposeful and consensual balancing act of respective interests in mutual welfare, against available resources. In favour of the power of the clinician, this asymmetrical relationship can be balanced by recognizing the clinician and patient as persons whose moral welfare counts equally, is interconnected and warrants equal consideration.

Among underlying problems here are patient-centred health care's disregard for the basic need to clarify the deep values of clinicians and patients and develop their character and shared motivation to act freely in ways that constitute personal flourishing, balanced welfare and the common good. Though exceptions to any principle are inevitable, the myriad exceptions to the principle of primacy of patient welfare indicate its inadequacy. And some of them are a perverse consequence of this inadequacy. For example, surgeons inappropriately avert risk when, fearing adverse consequences for themselves, as from the publication of patient death rates, they refuse to operate on patients at high risk of death despite full knowledge that operating is the patient's best or only chance of survival. To avoid this kind of exception, the motives of clinicians and patients must be made transparent and comprehensible.

Only then does it become widely possible to predict, explain and respond to actions by each party and the social institutions and structures to which their interactions give rise. Inattention by patient-centred health care to clinicians' and patients' character and motivation may help to explain why, after fifty years, this care model has not been widely implemented[14] and, for example, gives merely the illusion of challenging professional autonomy. How its processes relate to patient outcomes is poorly understood[15] and its track record is weak; its 'effects on patient satisfaction, health behaviour and health status are mixed'.[16] High patient satisfaction – for which the relationship with patient-centred health care appears strongest[15] – does not necessarily equate with experience of improvements in patient care and health outcomes.[17] In the United States the Patient-Centered Outcomes Research Institute has been funding researchers to conduct and disseminate comparative clinical effectiveness research to reveal the most effective patient-centred interventions. These interventions for patients mitigate patient-centred health care's neglect of science in health care but can be further developed because, for example, they are yet not compared with interventions that benefit patients *and* clinicians.

An independent inquiry recently published by the United Kingdom's Royal College of General Practitioners[18] nevertheless chose to retain usage of the term 'patient-centred' because this nomenclature is still 'commonly used across the health service, and is easily understood by both professionals and the public'. Patient-centred health care's credibility bears no causal relation to its frequency of use or clarity of meaning. But what is the alternative to patient-centred health care?

Unlike change leaders Paul Spiegelman and Britt Berrett – with whom I share concern for clinician welfare – I cannot recommend that '*Patients Come Second*'.[19] Their book encourages health care organizations to refocus their resources onto disengaged employees in order to reconnect them to the goal of enhancing the patient experience. However, expecting patients to benefit from employee engagement and self-care ignores the need of the more vulnerable moral agent – the patient – to benefit from care improvements directly, not merely indirectly through what looks like trickle-down theory. This theory, as encapsulated in the aphorism, 'a rising tide lifts all boats', may unnecessarily and inappropriately benefit clinicians – and whether it lifts patients, along with clinicians, depends on the nature of the 'tide'. An economic tide that boosts clinicians' incomes is unlikely to benefit patients. In contrast, if clinicians develop relational virtues like politeness, patients might well mirror this behaviour. So attention should be focused on how clinician welfare is grown and in order to safeguard against clinicians acting perversely in their own interests and providing inappropriate care.

Provision is needed for the direct, relational care of patients and clinicians functioning to support themselves and each other. Progress requires key stakeholders to have the wisdom and courage to act on this need. Leading professional and patient organizations worldwide – including the World Health Organization, World Medical Association and International Alliance of Patients' Organizations – have endorsed *person-centred health care*. However, despite these groups giving their imprimatur to this practice model, person-centred health care exhibits its own problems of early development.

Person-centred health care

The literature on person-centred health care has yet to define sufficiently well, and demonstrate clear agreement on, this model's meaning and scope. One consequence has been a common inability to understand how person-centred health care differs from patient-centred health care and what the linguistic shift promises. Indeed, literature on person-centred health care tends to misrepresent patient-centred health care. It creates a straw man when it misconstrues patient-centred health care as recipient-focused and patient-directed, rather than co-produced and patient-guided, and devalues how patient-centred health care already recognizes the patient as a person. So, when conceptualized to emphasize the personhood of only the patient, person-centred health care acts little differently from patient-centred care, re-dressing patient-centred health care in new clothes to bring the personhood of the patient to the fore. It is perhaps unsurprising therefore that person-centred health care has been identified as a type of patient-centred health care,[11] and many definitions of person-centred health care[20] are definitions of patient-centred health care. In these terms the new 'emperor [person-centred health care] has no clothes' that clearly differentiate it from patient-centred health care.

Such features only become evident once person-centred health care is conceptualized in a manner that heeds the World Health Organization's warning against confusing person-centred health care – which it calls 'people-centred care' – with patient-centred health care. The latter care, notes the World Health Organization, 'comprises an important part, but not the totality, of a people-centred approach'.[21] However, this public health arm of the United Nations has done little to directly distinguish the two care models, beyond locating people-centred health care in health systems that respond humanistically to the needs of individual people, families and communities. Failure to expose and recognize differences between person-centred (or people-centred) health care and patient-centred health care continues to squander opportunities inherent in person-centredness. So I find myself motivated to write this book to open up person-centred health care for detailed scrutiny in a manner that differentiates it from patient-centred health care, and then suggests what is needed to implement and review it.

The raison d'être of person-centred health care is not, as suggested by groups like the United Kingdom's Health Foundation,[22] to return control of health and health care to patients. From my perspective the imperative is to put first the person(s) of the patient and clinician, among others, in a person-to-person relationship of mutual, reciprocal engagement. This egalitarian perspective supports rather than compromises the wellness of clinicians to provide health care; motivates clinicians to pursue excellence through qualities of good character, such as pride in daily practice; and respects patients' capabilities to express their personhood by showing they care about their clinicians as well as themselves. These capabilities are important because, as persons, clinicians matter for their own sake and because when clinicians flourish as persons, patients flourish too. This book suggests that health care can move towards the ideal where clinicians and patients flourish as persons in a landscape whose moral contours elevate person-centred moments into person-centred cultures of practice.[23]

Book structure and style

This book takes a critical realist perspective of these issues. Assuming an objectively real world, which can only be provisionally understood, the book anatomizes them mainly for academics and postgraduate students engaged in learning, scholarship and research about person-centredness in health care and particularly medicine. In style the book is as much philosophical and literary as grounded in the health care sciences, and has two parts. Part I discusses the need to change how clinicians and patients interact in modern health care. Part II elaborates on the type of change needed – movement toward person-centred health care – and how to implement it and assess the progress that is made.

Part I, more specifically, discusses how renewed policy interest in patient-centred health care and other features of modern health systems undermine relational concern and respect for care of patients and clinicians as people and moral equals. To establish the *need for change*, Part I examines the clinician–patient relationship in terms of four directions of care: clinician to patient, clinician to self, patient to self, and patient to clinician. Chapters 2 to 5 focus respectively on each direction by speaking to challenges associated with the changing roles of clinician and patient in patient-centred health care. Collectively, the chapters indicate how patient-centred health care requires the clinician to care for patients before themselves. Patients can choose to care for themselves but are presumed unable or unneeded to care for the clinician as a person in a professional relationship in modern health systems.

Permeating Part I as a whole is my observation that the apparent obviousness of the principle of putting patient welfare first has discouraged its critical examination. Belief in this principle, including the implication that clinician welfare is secondary to helping patients, is suggested to be harming clinicians, patients and health system performance. Challenging a millennia-long focus solely on the patient, this thesis may surprise some readers. However, I am not the first person to question that the health profession really believes in putting patients' welfare first,[24] and to suggest that the principle of primacy of patient welfare is 'controversial at best, morally offensive at worst'.[25] Therefore my analysis will include appeals to the authority of expert others to garner visible and accountable open-mindedness, rather than epistemic trust in my critique of the principle of primacy of patient welfare.

Comprising Chapters 6 to 8, Part II develops my model of person-centred health care to demonstrate the kind of social change required to answer the previously discussed challenges. Putting the person, rather than embodied social roles, at the centre and 'heart' of health care, this model responds to needs and opportunities identified in Part I to balance the personal interests and welfare of patients and clinicians. Chapter 6 begins this task by sketching a bridge from patient-centred health care to person-centred health care. It sets out the concepts needed to envision person-centred health care; shows how this model is currently conceptualized much too broadly; and suggests, in turn, a new, generic definition of person-centred health care. Chapter 7 builds on this discussion. Suggesting a fundamental re-visioning of moral values in modern health care, the chapter deconstructs person-centred health care into seven defining values: flourishing, virtue, personalism, moral equality, pæanism, authenticity and consilience. Fundamental to distinguishing person-centred health care from patient-centred health care, these values are suggested to nourish together the roots of the care that entwine clinicians and patients in the directions explored by Chapters 2 to 5. The seven values link, in turn, to an ethic of virtue that brings to the fore considerations of the character, motivation and practice of the clinician and patient.

Advocacy of virtue can feel old-fashioned and conjure negative connotations like piety and righteousness. However, the virtues are not unappealing and unachievable qualities of moral saintliness. Although people may benefit from selfish behaviour, I denounce the Hobbesian anti-virtue bias encouraged by what began as the bad joke of Bernard Mandeville's *The Fable of the Bees*. Instead, I regard the virtues as character strengths that energize moral agents to practise good behaviour – just as they need regular exercise to improve their physical fitness – in response to moral demands of particular situations. This response is generally constitutive of an ideal middle path balanced between extremes of feeling. The path constructed by the virtues enables persons to act, and be trusted to act, consistently well in most circumstances for the right reasons. In so doing they can heal or alleviate problems and flourish. Grounded in a value-strong ethic of virtue, cultivating good character matters for its own sake and to rehumanize health care by making it person-centred.

Person-centred health care is the kind of health care that persons of virtue produce in order to be faithful to their moral values in facing moral dilemmas in health care – for example around cost-control and discordant expectations of patients and clinicians. In my Emergency Department example, I would have benefitted from exercising virtues like patience and gratitude for my health care. My physician and I might have benefitted from his demonstrating other virtues, such as humility and fortitude, by trusting in my illness narrative. We both could have prospered from practical wisdom in co-producing health care of shared benefit that synthesizes the sciences and humanities. As a scientific practice integrating caring and justice, the health care could then have enabled us each to flourish by maximizing our capabilities. This person-centred model shifts health care from a patient-centred, codified ethics of principle and duty-governed action for patient welfare and population health care.

Chapter 8 discusses what is needed to implement my framework as an integrated approach to balancing the welfare of patients and clinicians as persons, so they can thrive together. It advocates the civic theoretical and personalist perspective that persons are constitutive of communities. Resolving a potential tension between the individual and society, this perspective promotes social and political arrangements for creating cultural spaces in which persons can cultivate the virtues, promote mutuality and reciprocity, and actualize their capabilities to live a good and flourishing life. Focusing on the social conditions required for person-centred health care to generate and sustain such changes, the chapter discusses what is needed to realize lifelong opportunities for character development, including upbringing and education. It further considers the potential to develop and use emerging personal health technologies for purposes including moral bioenhancement. Lastly, it suggests how to indicate progress towards achieving person-centred health care that unifies character, social role and practice, and balances interests, virtues and moral norms within and between patients and clinicians.

Part II therefore presents a provocative statement of my understanding of what person-centred health care is, or at least how I believe it should be understood today. This understanding reflects my perspective as a non-clinician concerned equally with the welfare of patients and clinicians. I come to this project from an academic background of some 25 years, at the interface of the humanities, social sciences and health care. My work has progressively focused there on social theory and health care practice models including clinician–patient encounters. My insights also draw on my Jewish upbringing which embeds good practices in good character that continues to develop over a lifetime.

In this context my book offers a personal perspective in the hope that, although 'elephants are different to different people', readers will benefit from my own way of seeing the world in which what appears self-evident often is not. Yet, I strive not to be peremptory because, to be viable, no health system can be definitive and normatively prescriptive, particularly in relation to contested areas of social and moral life. Circumspection is needed because so much human knowledge is emergent, provisional and fallible. A sober implication of my discussion therefore is that the health care described in Chapter 5 as person-centred by others, does not necessarily or even usually fit my conceptualization. Nonetheless, debate about the nature, scope and significance of person-centred health care as a twenty-first century model is urgently needed and possible because person-centred health care is yet to progress toward a unified system of practice; and person-centred health care cannot be permitted to mean whatever people want. In these terms I advocate with passion for my reasoned advocacy for a value-based ethic of virtue.

Despite my relational focus on the clinician and patient, I often refer specifically to physicians to make clear that I am referring to medical care. However, this discussion is typically still relevant to clinicians in general. They include nurses and clinical pharmacists, as well as other members of the caring professions – including allied health professionals such as audiologists and dental hygienists – and related 'people professions' such as law, management and business.

The discussion is also germane to informal caregivers and family members who cannot be simply reduced to caregivers; and to hybridized, distributed roles such as clinician-managers. Increasingly moreover, health care is actually group-based or team-based – with patients contributing – rather than exclusively dyadic or paired. However, I wish to focus on the dyad because it is 'arguably the fundamental unit of interpersonal interaction and interpersonal relations',[26] even when it is embedded within larger social groups. Implicit in this focus is the non-independence and role distinguishability of the clinician and patient. I shall argue that erosion of distinguishability progressively weakens this dyad as an analytic construct but that reference to the shared personhood of the clinician and patient reassociates these roles.

My focus on person-centred clinical care is relevant in turn to 'people-centred public health'. Despite my considering the relationship between the clinician and patient – as persons – the concept of personhood avoids pitting individuals against aggregative structures like families and communities. Recognizing persons as relational by nature and constitutive of these social structures, person-centred health care distinguishes the person from the individual as an atomistic, biological organism and gives a unified account of human social life. Sociality continually emerges from, and is productive of, persons who strive within and beyond themselves to realize their capabilities to flourish.

Throughout the book, I will express the plural of 'person' sometimes as 'people' when I am not referring specifically to person-centred health care, but as 'persons' when I am discussing person-centred health care. I will also identify scholars by their full names on first use out of respect for their personhood. Lastly, in discussing person-centred health care, I must acknowledge my inadequacy in actualizing consistently the behaviour it commends. As a human being, I rarely achieve the ideals I aspire to reach, but progress toward them is a step towards excellence in health care and life. From this overview I invite you to consider my new conceptualization of person-centred health care.

References

1 Miles A, Mezzich J. Person-centered medicine: advancing methods, promoting implementation. *International Journal of Person Centered Medicine* 2011; 1: 423–8.

2 Bouckaert L, Leuven K. The project of a personalist economics. *Ethical Perspectives* 1999; 6: 20–33.

3 Hilton S. More human. *Designing a World Where People Come First*. London: WH Allen; 2015.

4 Sklansky M, Nadkarni N, Ramirez-Avila L. Banning the handshake from the health care setting. *Journal of the American Medical Association* 2015; 311: 2477–8.

5 Thomas L. *The Youngest Science: Notes of a Medicine-watcher*. New York: Bantam Books; 1983.

6 Vincent J. Give your patient a fast hug (at least) once a day. *Critical Care Medicine* 2005; 33: 1225–9.

7 Misselbrook D. Waving not drowning: virtue ethics in general practice. *British Journal of General Practice* 2015; 65: 226–7.

8 Ziegelstein R. Personomics. *JAMA Internal Medicine* 2015; 175: 888–9.

9 Albuquerque J, Deshauer D. Physician health: beyond work–life balance. *Canadian Medical Association Journal* 2014; 186: E502–3.

10 Chang A, Ritchie C. Patient-centered models of care: closing the gaps in physician readiness. *Journal of General Internal Medicine* 2015; 30: 870–2.

11 Tanenbaum S. What is patient-centered care? A typology of models and missions. *Health Care Analysis* 2015; 23: 272–87.

12 Shanafelt TD, Boone S, Tan L, Dyrbye L, Sotile W, Satele D, West C, Sloan J, Oreskovich M. Burnout and satisfaction with work–life balance among US physicians relative to the general US population. *Archives of Internal Medicine* 2012; 172: 1377–85.

13 Bardes CL. Defining 'patient-centered medicine'. *New England Journal of Medicine* 2012; 366: 782–3.

14 Fowler F, Gerstein B, Barry M. How patient centered are medical decisions? Results of a national survey. *JAMA Internal Medicine* 2013; 173: 1215–21.

15 Rathert C, Wyrwich MD, Boren SA. Patient-centered care and outcomes: a systematic review of the literature. *Medical Care Research and Review* 2013; 70: 351–79.

16 Dwamena F, Holmes-Rovner M, Gaulden CM, Jorgenson S, Sadigh G, Sikorskii A, Lewin S, Smith RC, Coffey J, Olomu A. Interventions for providers to promote a patient-centred approach in clinical consultations. *Cochrane Database of Systematic Reviews* 2012; 12: CD003267; doi:10.1002/14651858.

17 Kupfer J, Bond E. Patient satisfaction and patient-centered care. Necessary but not equal. *Journal of the American Medical Association* 2012; 308: 139–40.

18 Royal College of General Practitioners. *An Inquiry into Patient Centred Care in the 21st Century*. London: Royal College of General Practitioners; 2014.

19 Spiegelman P, Berrett B. *Patients Come Second. Leading Change by Changing the Way You Lead*. New York: An Inc. Original; 2013.

20 Entwistle V, Watt I. Treating patients as persons: using a capabilities approach to support delivery of person-centred care. *American Journal of Bioethics* 2013; 13: 29–39.

21 World Health Organization (WHO). *People at the Centre of Health Care: Harmonising Mind and Body, People and Systems*. Geneva: WHO; 2007.

22 de Silva, D. for The Health Foundation. *Helping Measure Person-centred Care. Evidence Review*. London: The Evidence Centre; 2014.

23 McCormack B, McCance T. *Person-centred Nursing: Theory and Practice*. Oxford: Wiley-Blackwell; 2010.

24 Gillon R. 'The patient's interests always come first'? Doctors and society. *British Medical Journal* 1986; 292: 398–400.

25 Veatch R. Character formation in professional education: a word of caution. In: Kenny N, Shelton W, editors. *Lost Virtue (Advances in Bioethics, Volume 10)*. Bingley: Emerald Group Publishing 2006; pp. 29–45.

26 Kenny D, Kashy D, Cook W. *Dyadic Data Analysis*. New York: Guilford Press; 2006.

Part I

The need for change

2 Clinician care of the patient

Introduction

Health care systems depend heavily on the delivery of patient care by clinicians, including physicians and other qualified health care professionals. Patient 'care' is used here as a portmanteau term describing values and technical and interpersonal practices by clinicians.[1] Technical performance relates to their service provision for patient welfare, whilst interpersonal behaviour adds concerned attention – that is, caring – for patient welfare. I intend to convey both meanings in mapping the myriad factors that blunt the ability of patient-centredness to provide health care to patients. The chapter begins by defining patient centred health care and critically discussing core features of its historical and contemporary landscape, including a commitment to moral principles of health care professionalism such as primacy of patient welfare. I then discuss how four sets of characteristics of modern health care are testing clinicians' professional commitment and ability to implement this principle, among others, in order to practise patient-centred health care – on whose 'watch' the challenges to this care model have been permitted to expand. The result is an unmet need for health systems to improve the organization and delivery of clinician care for patient welfare. In common with Chapters 3 to 5, this chapter underpins my discussion of the need for person-centred health care in Part II of the book.

Patient-centred health care

To understand patient-centred health care, look at Figure 2.1. It depicts a lithograph painted by the Norwegian artist, Edvard Munch. What I notice first when viewing this image is the large face of a man in the foreground. His wide eyes stare at me; tormented eyes that call attention to themselves; searching eyes – set within an isolated, dark, compact face. They gaze away from the human figures standing behind him, figures petitioning relief. Beyond the large face, these figures in the mid-ground comprise a half-disrobed woman who coquets with a dark-clothed man. Her gaze and fine threads of her hair bind them together, as if into one. They stand beneath a giant tree that I perceive to be the tree of life framed by a symbol of creative suffering, the 'flower of pain'. To me

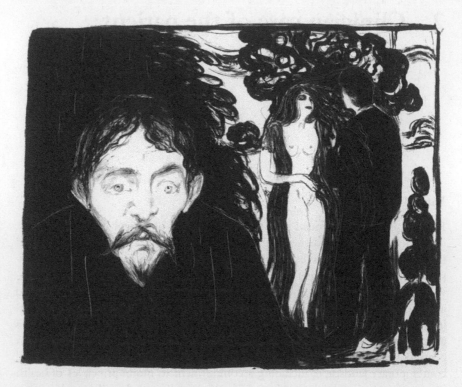

Figure 2.1 Edvard Munch, *Jealousy,* 1896 (source: photograph of original piece courtesy
of Imaging Department © President and Fellows of Harvard College. Reproduced with kind permission from Harvard Art Museums/Fogg Museum, Gift
of Lynn G. Straus in memory of Philip A. Straus, 2012.266).

this composition is intended to be partly out of balance in order to bring
together a hierarchy of design elements that create dramatic tension and cause
discomfort. All the elements add visual weight to my use of the image as a metaphor of patient-centred health care – which overall is likewise unbalanced.

For me the metaphor draws on how differentiating light from shadow
exposes what the subjects of the image can see or not; where sight substitutes
metonymically for care. Pushed forward, yet hidden in shadow, the outsized
male face signifies a clinician in distress. The woman and man who stand in the
light represent patients, who appear self-entranced. Illuminating their welfare,
the light bathing the patients allows them to see themselves and develop a sense
of knowing inclusive of the rational order of the 'En-light-enment' and of what
is important for them to care about. To the extent that their visibility exposes
them as human subjects in need of caring, these patients can self-care and be
cared for by others, including the clinician; at least if he were to turn around
and find them within his sight. The French verb, *regarder,* encapsulates this dual
capacity to look at and feel concern.

In the darkness defined by the light shining on the patients, the clinician cannot see himself in order to self-care. Nor can his patients easily see him and care for him. The shroud of darkness over the clinician disembodies his visible presence to them as a person and moral subject, who needs to self-care and receive from others – including patients – the care they can freely offer him. The clinician's self-care and capability to receive patient care have become subordinated therefore to his care of them as patients who present their bodies in the light for unobscured treatment. Indeed the shadow over the clinician heightens attention to the lit presence of the patients. Redolent of Simon Peter in the New Testament, the shadow of the clinician touches them healingly. For their good, the clinician surrenders his own interests; he is like Odin, the supreme Nordic deity who sacrificially suspended himself from the tree of life. Most simply however, the clinician in the dark can potentially see and care for illuminated patients who can self-care but cannot see him in order to reciprocate care.

Likewise, patient-centred health care is an ideal that expects modern clinicians to focus attention on, and care for, patients rather than themselves. Putting patients at the centre of health care, this model explicates patients' capacity to be active participants who, beyond receiving health care, can see and care for themselves but not really see or care for their clinicians. The person of the clinician, even when in front of patients' eyes, may not be clearly perceived, at least as a person; and the role of clinician may be poorly understood. Therefore, the model illuminates patients who partner with the 'unseen' clinician to help care for their own welfare. Broadly speaking, this shared care of the patient 'is respectful of and responsive to individual patient preferences, needs, and values and [ensures] that patient values guide all clinical decisions'.[2] Widely considered the standard for interpersonal clinical care, its normative commitment to care first and foremost for the patient has its ethical roots in the oath historically sworn to by physicians and attributed to the ancient Greek physician, Hippocrates of Cos.

Most contemporary oaths sworn by medical students vary significantly from the Hippocratic Oath, which nevertheless stands as the founding document for western medical ethics. In its original form, it is religious. Under the protection of the divinities, it requires physicians to commit to living a 'pure' life and providing rational medical care to patients as their primary duty in the healing tradition of the deity of medicine, Asklepios. Patients are represented in the Oath as passive bearers of sickness, whose origin is physical and who depend largely on the beneficence and humanity of the physician to treat them. In caring for patients the secular physician – a word deriving from the Greek term for nature, *physis* – perceived the body to function as an integrated whole in a law-governed natural order.

Therefore, Greek medicine as a profession was holistic. Presuming the unity of the body, mind and behaviour, this view was universalized from the Middle Ages into early modern times. The medical profession then looked for new ways to understand and manage sickness as a shift in the sites of production of medical knowledge took place from classical learning and bedside medicine to hospital medicine.[3-5] The last development in the age of Enlightenment embraced the use of the scientific method, which introduced options that might improve health outcomes for patients but also distanced them from physicians. Constructed as a mechanical body in clinical medicine, the patient became a passive product of the medical gaze. The physician used disease-centred thinking to manage the patient's problem – defined in reductionist, biological terms – to promote the patient's health. It was not until the mid-1960s, some 2,500 years after Hippocrates, that principle-based moral theories began to reshape this ethic of beneficence. Despite a continuing commitment to contribute to the welfare of the patient, medicine and health care then progressively demonstrated a new respect particularly for patient autonomy and patient rights. Epitomizing this development, the model of patient-centred health care, as we have come to know it, achieved deep respect for patients as people. It recognized patients as embodied and autonomous subjects functioning in the everyday world they experience. Yet, beneficence continued to constitute the main purpose of medicine and health care.

The British psychoanalysts, Michael Balint[6] and his wife Enid Balint,[7] first described patient-centred health care as 'whole person-centred medicine'.[8] Settling on the term 'patient-centred care', they provided a method to help clinicians manage patients' psychological and relational problems, as well as physical illness. Patient-centred health care further evolved with the development of principles of family medicine, for example by Frans Huygen during the late 1970s in the Netherlands,[9] and was formally developed from the mid-1980s by Joseph Levenstein and family medicine scholars at Canada's University of Western Ontario.[10,11] Becoming the standard for patient–clinician communication, their clinical method of patient-centred interviewing[12] provided a simple way for clinicians to implement and validate George Engel's complementary model of biopsychosocial care.[13] To recognize the whole person of the patient, Engel's model corrected the reductionism of the biomedical model by integrating understanding and management of biological, psychological and social influences on health and disease. The patient-centred clinical method also responded to patients' explanatory models of illness[14] vis-à-vis the clinician's disease-centred understanding and clinician-centred care. It drew on the narrative competence of the clinician[15] to elicit and understand patients' values and the meaning of their illness experience in the context of their life stories. It further sought to inform and be responsive to patients' preferences, as an intrinsic goal of health care, by involving patients as active participants in health care, for example through shared decision-making. Definitions of patient-centred health care have continued to develop, moving discussion of this care beyond the patient–clinician relationship to health care institutions but continuing to emphasize the experience of the patient who can co-produce care with the clinician across health care settings.[16]

In the United States, work on clinician–patient communication and shared decision-making has built on this pedigree of patient-centredness, contributing in 2001 to the Institute of Medicine[17] recognizing patient-centred care as an explicit aim of high quality health care. As a rule for redesigning its health system, the Institute stipulated that 'The patient is the source of control.' The vague but radical nature of this rule may help to explain why the meaning of patient-centred health care is still debated. Aspirationally however, the rule speaks to a need widely recognized internationally to respect lay values, experience and preferences in health care. Patients and the public have traditionally lacked the power to shape health services, yet recent participatory initiatives in many health systems include these groups in designing, implementing and evaluating system improvements to the safety, functionality and useability of health care. The improvements reflect renewed policy interest in the principles of patient-centred health care,[18] most saliently in the United States where they help to arrest decline in primary care through system-wide change under the Patient Protection Affordable Care Act (PPACA).[19] Reforms at the federal and state levels are integrating patient-centred concepts into health care standards through service delivery innovations like the patient-centred medical home. This team-based philosophy aims to transform physician-led primary care practices into cost-effective organizations to enhance patient engagement and experience and population health. To achieve these aims the homes coordinate and integrate comprehensive care and a whole person emphasis across the health system. Moot however is whether patient-centred health care includes population health care or sits uneasily with it.[20]

Indeed, controversy still characterizes the fundamental goal of patient-centred health care. Even its own proponents question whether this model is important either for its own sake, regardless of its impact, or as a means of improving the quality of patient care. If the latter goal is accepted, the ability of patient-centred health care to achieve it has still not been clearly demonstrated. Mixed results have been reported overall for relationships between patient-centred health care and clinical outcomes,[21] and no encouragement comes from recent United States findings on the effectiveness of patient-centred medical homes in improving the quality, utilization and costs of modern health care.[22] What makes patient-centred health care 'morally right' has received little scholarly attention.[23]

Principles

From my perspective, the most cogent moral justification for patient-centred health care is that it reflects ethical norms of inherent value, as exemplified by statements of bioethical principles for health care professionalism.[24] Prominent among these statements is the 2002 Physician Charter.[25] Produced by leaders of internal medicine across the United States and Europe, and subsequently endorsed by more than 130 professional organizations worldwide, the Charter has been suggested to be even more relevant today than when it was developed.[26] Its 'action agenda' for elucidating and raising the profile of medical professionalism has stimulated physicians to reassert their authority in collaborating with other professionals to resist external challenges to medical care.

These challenges have arisen because 'medical practice is embedded in a health care system that determines the content and scope of professional autonomy'.[27] This system produces tribalism between clinician specialities and clinicians and managers who expect clinicians to achieve targets for excellence and quality improvement amid growing health care costs, resource constraints, technological change and external regulation. Also demanding action are policy expectations for physicians to help reduce inequalities in health care and promote social justice through individualized care in the context of population health goals.

The Charter explicates the need for physicians to implement three moral principles of medical care; and clinical care more generally. These principles – primacy of patient welfare, patient autonomy and social justice – align with the commitment of patient-centred health care to: put patient welfare first; have due regard for, and facilitate, patients' autonomous decision-making; and promote fairness in patients' access to health care. Shared alike by professionalism and patient-centred health care, the principles reformulate similar moral norms that are included in some form, on the basis of a common morality, in other classical ethical frameworks like rule-based deontology. Indeed, the prima facie principles – which can directly conflict – guide the local formulation of more specific rules and obligations. From the principles, the Charter has derived ten professional responsibilities (or 'commitments') whose contractual language gives it a legalistic tone. These responsibilities expose patient-centred health care as a duty-based ethic centred on patient welfare. I want to discuss the principle of primacy of patient welfare and then challenges to it from inside and outside the Charter.

As the centrepiece of patient-centred health care, the principle of primacy of patient welfare declares that the welfare needs of the patient are paramount. There has been a continuing and widespread reluctance to question this moral principle as a fundamental tenet of health care professionalism and even as a moral requirement for clinical care. The burden of proving the rightness of the principle and, therefore, of patient-centred health care itself has fallen on the commentators who favour something else.[23] The principle has appeared self-evidently right because patients have greater immediate health care needs than clinicians, and health care by definition is a form of beneficence. Moreover, favouring the clinician, a structural imbalance of power 'in the form of knowledge, skills, access to resources, social authorization, and legal legitimation'[28] requires patients to trust their clinician to put their patients' welfare above clinician self-interest. For such reasons physicians swear publicly to the Hippocratic Oath or more commonly some similar oath such as the Declaration of Geneva (Physicians Oath) when they graduate from medical school. As a counterpoint to the Ring of Gyges myth in the Second Book of Plato's, *The Republic*, they swear to honour the expectation of fidelity to patients.

Although the oath taking is most often ceremonial and non-obligatory, a social contract is now widely believed to entitle people to receive health (care) as a human right; and the patient–clinician encounter also frequently entails a legal contract for service. Clinicians are professionals paid to exercise their special body of knowledge and skills in the best interests of those they serve; and in so doing benefit themselves, for example through income, status and satisfaction. On top of these reasons, health care is a moral enterprise, not merely a scientific or business one, committed to professional integrity and arguably to selfless altruism. Within the realm of moral and professional duty therefore, clinicians act to support patients' health and healing; and, stretching health care's morality, they may also offer patients and society contested benefits like genetic testing and reproductive controls.

In this context the primacy of patient welfare underscores health care professionalism and health policy developments worldwide. Today, for example, the publicly funded National Health Service of the United Kingdom explicitly requires clinicians to put the interests of patients ahead of their own.[29] Regardless of who is expected to benefit more from having their interests satisfied, this principle guides the application of levers of choice and competition to improve health services. Another argument for putting patient welfare first is that problems arise not when clinician welfare is put second but when clinicians fail to receive a minimum, sufficient level of care. However, a problem with this claim is that providing care that is merely sufficient and hence satisfactory or 'good enough' is not necessarily in the best interests of the patient or the clinician. Good enough tends to act against achieving the best, the best requiring optimizing the welfare of both the patient and the clinician.

Challenges

There are many exceptions, moreover, to the principle of primacy of patient welfare. From an informal survey of the literature, David Wendler[30] documented 27 widely acknowledged exceptions to physicians acting in the best interests of the present patient. The exceptions come from: competing claims, for example for physician self-care; other patients; and family members as well as society. Such exceptions highlight limits to the resources – including the time and power – of physicians to know and be responsive to each patient's health interests[31] compared with the public good, their own moral interests as physicians, and the interests of other patients and family members. Wendler's[30] concern lies less with the principle of primacy of patient welfare, to which exceptions require a 'compelling justification', than with the need, he perceived, to establish an oversight authority that could provide systematic guidance on which exceptions are legitimate and how to manage them. Yet, the exceptions he identified speak to the complexity of the principle and cast doubt on whether the medical profession, and health professionals more generally, truly believe and practise it. Thirty years ago Ranaan Gillon[32] expressed similar doubt by stating that if the medical profession 'really believed that the patient's interests always come first, then it presumably would not allow medical time and effort to be diverted away from direct therapeutic activity'. Reinforcing this scepticism has been a continuing, general failure by physicians to hold each other to a best-interest standard.

I wish to suggest four sets of challenges to the primacy of *patient* welfare as a properly sufficient concern of modern health care. The Charter itself highlights the first set of challenges that come .from potential conflict with the principles of respect for patient autonomy and social justice. Second, the concept of patienthood is losing specificity and clear differentiation as a meaningful category. Third, challenges arise from recognizing health (care) as a human right, not specifically a patient right, and its growing reconstruction within health systems as a 'commodified right'. Lastly I will suggest how recent attempts to view dehumanization as potentially functional act inadvertently against patient welfare. The overall discussion challenges the nature and scope of patient-centred health care.

1 The Physician Charter

Though designed to resist health system changes and other forces 'tempting physicians to abandon their commitment to the principle of primacy of patient welfare',[33] the Charter itself risks compromising this principle. The principle of primacy of patient welfare is set against other moral principles with which it can conflict. The Charter first invites consideration of how to reconcile the conflict that can arise between patient autonomy and physician concern for patient welfare. When there is conflict, then even with deliberation and judgement there will be gains and losses for patient-centred health care: either patient welfare triumphs, which undermines respect for patient autonomy as a feature of patient-centred health care, or else patient autonomy weakens physicians' benevolent concern for patient welfare. Second, a tension can develop between social justice and patient welfare. The Charter effectively divides physician loyalties to individual patients vis-à-vis society as a whole, without explaining how to manage the conflicts within a functional alliance with society.[34] Let us consider the various challenges posed by respect for patient autonomy and social justice respectively.

Respect for patient autonomy

Respect for the autonomy of patients – or, as Tom Delbanco and his colleagues[35] have expressed this principle, 'nothing about me without me' – implies the need of physicians and other clinicians to safeguard patients' informed agency and full involvement in decision-making about their health care. Clinicians are expected to enable patients to share decisions that are faithful to these patients' values and preferences. However, disagreement over the precise meaning, scope and moral significance of respect for this principle is problematic when there is no standard clinical choice to make – such as whether to screen routinely for prostate cancer or treat early stages of this disease. It is unknown in this situation what best serves the patient's welfare, which necessitates comparing different options, mindful that the option preferred by the patient may differ from the option that the clinician favours.

Consistent with political movements for civic and human rights and liberal individualism, recent decades have witnessed patients' growing competence and agency to make the final choice from options available to them for their health care, even when this choice does not maximize their welfare. Indeed, clinicians commonly stretch patients' competence to choose how to proceed because, grounded in personal dignity, patient autonomy has intrinsic rather than necessarily instrumental worth, for example in promoting welfare or quality of life. Clinicians who promote patients' autonomy appeal to patients to become more self-directed[36] and, in some versions of patient-centred health care, to control decision-making.[2,37] Mandatory patient decision-making has been advocated mainly because patients alone directly experience the consequences of decisions made about their health care.[38] In turn, amid increasing complexity in modern health care, clinicians might have no preference or be truly uncertain as to which clinical option to recommend. They may also wish to share responsibility for risks associated with the decision taken, while wanting to minimize third party regulation of the content of health care. However, clinicians may effectively restrict the ability of patients to express autonomy.

Clinicians understand that illness can burden and distract patients, who may also lack in their individual circumstances the intellectual and emotional capabilities and other resources needed to make and implement choices that promote their welfare. Moreover, patients cannot know what information they want disclosed to them until they know it. Too much information may increase their decision-making autonomy but inappropriately frighten them and reduce their welfare. For such reasons, clinicians may communicate poor prognoses to patients in hopeful terms, which patients may perceive as compassionate.[39] In this environment, patients may not always want and be able to make informed health care decisions, alone or even with their clinician. Therefore, most clinicians are wary of mandatory patient decision-making that can leave patients feeling overwhelmed, isolated and abandoned. Shared decision-making offers both parties a compromise between patient autonomy and patient welfare, and provides scope for clinicians to explain to patients why they cannot always have what they request. Requiring clinicians to do what the patient wants – such as to receive an antibiotic for a viral infection – can act against the welfare of the patient, others or both, at least in the long term. As Robert Veatch[40] has stated, 'Giving each of one's patients everything that could benefit them would not only be immoral, but is actually illegal when it commands resources rightfully belonging to others.' Similarly, a need to protect the public health may require clinicians to oppose particular preferences of the patient, as exemplified by a statutory duty to notify certain infectious diseases.

Consequently, not only is patient autonomy frequently optional in clinical practice but clinicians may restrict information giving to patients and be reluctant to let patients' 'irrational' choices trump their own clinical understanding of what best serves patients' welfare.[41] Drawing on the principle of therapeutic privilege and despite digital democratization of health information, clinicians therefore continue to act as gatekeepers to personalized health care information. They offer individual patients the information that, in their judgement, is clinically reasonable to give them. This information will enable these patients to pursue safely and conscientiously their personal health goals, while serving the good of others. Clinicians may further influence patient decision-making by limiting patients' treatment options. Patient autonomy here tends to function as a negative right since patients cannot usually expect to receive whatever treatments they want. Patients can at best accept or reject the treatments their clinician offers them. These treatment options may depend on whether preferences that patients have expressed fit with clinicians' knowledge of these patients' deep values – and hence seem authentic and truly autonomous.[42] On balance, the growth of patient agency dilutes the autonomy of the clinician to protect patient welfare, despite leaving it mostly intact.[43] In other words, patient welfare still tends to trump patient autonomy as a feature of patient-centred health care.

Social justice

The principle of social justice acts as a brake on the principles of primacy of patient welfare and respect for patient autonomy by reflecting how patient-centred health care has expanded its focus on personal health care to include (individualized) population health care. However, there is a risk of overstating this transition, since concern for population health has been evident for millennia. It is sometimes stated that the Hippocratic corpus obliges physicians to care for their patients, without concern for distributive justice,[44] yet in Greek society the concept of the individual patient was indivisible from the population. Today this notion still characterizes communitarian discourse – saliently among indigenous peoples such as New Zealand Māori, for whom 'Individual identity exists within whānau [extended family] and is indivisible from whānau.'[45] Nevertheless, for most people living in the West, the individual and society signify separate but interrelated social realms.

Success in bridging these realms has proved elusive. Recent decades have looked to patient-centred health care to repair the schism that took place a century ago between clinical health care – characterized by its focus on the individual patient – and community-oriented public health.[46] The 1978 Alma Ata Declaration[47] laid down some of the tenets of patient-centred health care, such as health promotion for all, which resonate with the drive of the Physician Charter and, as noted above, with other reforms that have been introduced to provide population health care in countries like the United States.[48] However, expecting clinicians to exercise stewardship of scarce societal resources weakens their ability to meet their fiduciary responsibility to put first the welfare of the present patient. Primary care clinicians, for example, are commonly expected to promote routine screening tests such as mammography even though these tests may benefit the community more than most participating patients.[49] Hence, the Physician Charter can cast clinicians unreasonably as 'double agents'.[50]

Contrary to the Charter's claim, health care has no 'contract with society', which can form the foundation of principles and responsibilities for health care professionalism. In creating such a contract by moving professionalism from a covenantal model to one prescribing clinician responsibilities in contractual language, the Charter signals distrust of key values of clinicians, such as beneficence – and arguably therefore puts patients second.[51,52] Put simply, the Charter constructs a model of population health care which can lose sight of the welfare of individual patients. The Munch painting, *Spring Evening on Karl Johan Street*, is emblematic of this consuming process. A lone, shadow-covered man walks past the life-frightened, moon-faced people who 'sleepwalk' past him. So brightly lit are their pallid faces that their individuality is lost within the compressed file of solitary figures. In the same way, population health care over-illuminates patients as individuals, who can appear almost indistinguishable from the background population, from each other and from their clinician. It is as if the over-illuminated patients can be imagined to fuse in the approaching light.

I have been focusing thus far on social justice in distributing health care to the whole population and to individual patients in the light of population-based goals. However, the principle of social justice also indicates a need to treat clinicians fairly in allocating health care resources. Health systems, including clinicians and patients, have an interest in caring about the welfare of clinicians as much as patients (Chapters 4 and 5) and hence in putting persons or people first, rather than merely patients (Part II). Nevertheless, qualifying this discussion is the growing porosity of the terms 'patient' and 'clinician', which reduces the meaningfulness of principles such as primacy of patient welfare.

2 Erosion of meaningful difference

The concept of the patient appears straightforwardly to signify the social actor playing the role of receiving health care. However, this semblance of simple meaning belies complexity. Retaining the trace of an individual who is under health care, the concept of the patient has become stretched to overlap related concepts like 'population' and even 'clinician' within grey zones whose boundaries themselves are uncertain. Not only does role convergence characterize clinicians and modern patients but also modern society increasingly views all people as patients requiring health care. Even though these patients have never been healthier than they are now, health systems construct them more and more as sick. Moreover, as more epidemiology is put into clinical practice, patients are managed alike. The result of such developments, stated the sociologist Jean Baudrillard, is 'a viral loss of determinacy ... [and] confusion of types',[53] which weakens the case for privileging the welfare of patients as a special group. Let us consider how everyone has become a patient and how this role obscures the personhood of patients. Clinicians, moreover, tend to treat alike these patients who increasingly resemble clinicians in ways that patient-centred health care struggles, by definition, to accommodate.

All people are becoming patients

Forty years ago, Marshall Marinker[54] observed that clinicians create patients, and certainly the answer to the question, 'What is a patient?' has changed over time. From the Latin *patiens*, the word patient originally denoted a person who suffers or bears a burden. The term, *patient*, still echoes this meaning of 'one who is acted upon' in patiently tolerating clinical care. However, this meaning has expanded. Beyond a focus on, and orientation toward, the family as a unit of care in family medicine, society itself has been transformed into a kind of patient. Moving beyond the generation when a person could be sick without becoming a patient,[54] all of its members have become patients linked by risk assessment and control. At the same time the over-brightness of the light of population health care has reduced the contrast between sick patients and others. Through increasing medicalization of human conditions and problems, this light has made sick patients difficult to distinguish from healthy persons – who traditionally have not been considered patients – and from the population as a whole.

Stated simply therefore, everyone today is a patient to the extent that patients no longer comprise only those who are sick or are worried they are sick. Patients also include those with no pathology. Society has encouraged them to restructure their everyday routines and increase clinical contact to reduce their risk of developing serious disease, improve their health and provide profitable markets for health care as an industry. As David Morris explained, health has become 'too important to be wasted on people who are perfectly well ... [and] happens not so much in the absence of illness as in its presence'.[55] In this context, family carers have become 'hidden patients' whose stresses and health needs often lack visibility. Moreover, as 'wounded healers', even clinicians have become patients.

Stretching the meaning of patienthood in this manner cannot fully extinguish the meaning of the patient as a person who has established 'a healing relationship with another who articulates society's willingness and capacity to help'.[54] However, especially within patient-centred primary health care, a powerful movement toward preventive medicine, including health promotion, has shifted clinicians' attention, 'from the sick to the well, from the old to the young and from the poor to the rich'.[56] To be precise, the transition in health service delivery has been less from the sick to the well than from the sick to the quasi-sick. It has been towards socially constructing increasing proportions of the population, who feel well, as simultaneously and apparently sick – for example on the basis of barely abnormal test results. In these terms not only is everyone a patient but also everyone is sick. This shift reflects the medicalization of all aspects of human life, including mood and lifestyle behaviour such as food choices. Just as Gustav Klimt's panel, *Medicine*, depicts Hygieia as a symbol of seduction, so too has medicalization seduced modern society and its clinician agents into over-focusing on health and expanding health care markets. In at least four ways, medicalization persists in Western society.

First, experiences that this society once considered a normal part of human adult life – such as sex and pregnancy – now commonly attract medical attention and intervention. Medicalization of symptoms has spawned diagnoses of new medical disorders like female sexual arousal disorder, and has created profitable opportunities to market new treatments. Moreover, the medical gaze has widened from signs and symptoms of illness to risk factors as spaces of possibility of illness. These risk factors are sometimes presented as preconditions or subclinical conditions among 'pre-vivors'. All social spheres have witnessed this growth of surveillance and control by the medical gaze on the population, for example through public health campaigns and screening. Michel Foucault's concept of 'indefinite medicalization' signifies how social and normalizing functions of this gaze impose themselves on populations without responding to the interests and demands of individual patients.

Second, the proportion of the population documented to have existing disease has swollen. For marginal gains, people have been increasingly diagnosed as having one or more of a range of diseases including hypertension, hyperlipidaemia and diabetes. Physicians may diagnose disease and predict clinical benefit (or harm) of treatment on the basis of surrogate endpoints or biomarkers, such as low-density lipoprotein (LDL) cholesterol concentrations. Thus, the biomarkers have become new disease entities. Ever-lower, arbitrary thresholds have been set in place by clinical guidelines and applied to these measures that ostensibly distinguish people with disease from others without the condition. Yet, the LDL cholesterol concentration is not, in itself, a reliable surrogate for cardiovascular benefit.

Third, if people cannot be meaningfully categorized into those who either do or do not have, say, hyperlipidaemia or high blood pressure, everyone has these conditions to some degree. And irrespective of the levels of individual risk factors for vascular disease events, the people at elevated total risk of these events may benefit from treatment, for example with low-cost statins, without experiencing serious adverse effects.[57] One implication is 'Statins for all by the age of 50 years?'[58] By then the event risk begins to warrant the clinician and patient discussing (absolute) risks and benefits of drug treatment (especially with movement in the United States[59] to initiate the most effective statin treatment rather than titrate statin use to reach LDL cholesterol targets). A polypill combining low doses of different medicines has also been proposed when risk factors for vascular disease are only slightly abnormal. Yet, since life is a terminal condition, healthy low risk can never be healthy enough. Whether millions of healthy people are best served by medicating them is still debated.

Moreover, arguably the greatest loss in people's lives is not their physical death, but their loss of quality of life, including what dies inside them when they dwell too much on – and try to control – the risk of becoming sick. What can die is their ability to accept risks inherent in life and live in enjoyment and equanimity with their human limitations and finitude. So long as healthy people without disease remain trapped by fear, whether irrational or rational, they will continue to divert some resources for clinical care away from the sickest people.

Population health care rings this bell of anxiety even though, while the population as a whole can be expected to benefit, some patients are harmed and most patients derive little, if any, personal benefit from preventive care (the 'prevention paradox').

Fourth, despite the continuing primacy of Hippocrates' injunction on clinicians to 'do no harm', applying clinical knowledge through diagnosis and treatments can cause illness, as an unintended side effect. Some harm is unavoidable. Statins, for example, commonly produce side effects like joint pain. Nevertheless, even major 'harm' can benefit patients as exemplified by surgery performed as an act of 'calculated violence'. Other patient harm can result from health care interventions that are unnecessary or, worse, inappropriate. For example, consider potentially dangerous side effects of the pharmaceutical treatment of the increasing number of children diagnosed with the Attention Deficit and Hyperactivity Disorder (ADHD). These side effects are empirical and, beyond the medical history, are not predictable for specific individuals. Hence, uncertainty compounds the clinical risk of iatrogenesis. So too does the possibility that pathology motivates treatment of ADHD with stimulant medication. Rather, the key aims of treatment are to reduce symptoms and improve normalcy, function and performance within certain social, including educational, settings. Iatrogenesis results also from public health interventions in groups of individuals, which returns us to the notion of the ever-narrowing distinction between individual patients and groups they constitute in the population.

Patienthood can mask personhood

While everyone is becoming a patient, the totalizing term, *patient*, struggles to accommodate the diverse meanings that lay people may attach to their role in health care. Some individual patients do not want to be described as patients – on whom health care can be centred. People who have been diagnosed with conditions including inflammatory bowel disease[60] and Parkinson's disease commonly do not refer to themselves as patients or want others to call them patients. From their perspective, a designation of patienthood reduces them to their disease and is inconsistent with their *personhood*, including their active ability to participate in an informed manner and with autonomy in decision-making about their health care. 'People-*first* language' is further evident in the disability field. The term 'people with disabilities' rather than 'disabled people' puts people's personhood ahead of their disabilities and describes what they have, not who they are. Even though, by emphasizing a lack of ability, 'disability' itself is detractory, the shift in language resists the primacy of welfare of the patient and facilitates a re-scoping of the social role of the patient in modern health care. Exemplifying this recalibration are increased sharing and democratization of health information through participatory infrastructures like the Open Growth platform of Sage Bionetworks' Real Names Discovery Pilot. Many people nevertheless remain content to be described as patients when they receive health care. At the same time they illustrate how it is not necessarily true that

'The sick, whom we profess to treat, are vulnerable, anxious, and dependent.'[61] Though it has become commonplace to describe patients as suffering from medical conditions like diabetes, patients may or may not experience suffering – as a severe, negative threat of discomfort or pain on their conscious intactness.

Certainly, most of the patients who are *not* ill do not suffer from being patients, although some of them do. Of the patients who experience discomfort from illness, some do not suffer as a result, despite others commonly equating this discomfort with suffering. Other ill patients do suffer from their condition, sometimes terribly. Their suffering may manifest in physical symptoms or in feeling abandoned, alone or in despair. Although culturally shaped, their suffering is personal. No less an attribute of personhood than patienthood, it constitutes an insufficient basis for patient-centred health care that puts the welfare of patients ahead of all persons. I want to elaborate on the notions that suffering is not distinctive to patients and can even be useful, and indeed necessary, for healing.

Some patients come to feel at ease with – or despite – their illness. Non-life-threatening illness might not worsen any suffering they experience for other reasons, like awareness of finitude as a condition of human life. Their illness therefore might not burden them; and not mandate primacy of welfare. The English poet, John Keats used the term 'negative capabilities' to describe this kind of openness to all human experience. And with this receptiveness, patients may experience illness as a 'good enough' part of what they can reasonably expect from their human life – a life that has been gifted to them, a life that is not death and for which they may feel grateful compared with other persons worse off than they. Hence, illness is not experienced as suffering in the light of this personal meaning.[62] Even patients who do not accept their illness may feel anger more than suffering and reassert autonomy.[63]

When patients do suffer, their suffering, like that of clinicians and family care-givers, can easily go unrecognized. When illness adds to suffering, this experience is not necessarily bad. A Jewish Midrash (Rabbinic commentary) states that until the time of Jacob, people died in the absence of illness. God granted Jacob's prayer for the *gift* of illness so that people could prepare for their death. Christian theology goes further in suggesting that people cannot complete living and become fully human painlessly or without suffering.[64] C.S. Lewis,[65] for example, drew on personal experience to explain that pain, even when producing resentment as a form of suffering, can facilitate personal growth and bring out the best in persons. Shakespeare had illustrated how such development can take place. In *King Lear*, Lear and Gloucester suffer from their wrongs but, through their suffering, find some moral redemption. Their suffering catalysed their acquiring virtues like insight, humility and humanity. Though suffering can also be destructive and meaningless, in combination with virtues such as hope and faith, it can be endured by people who feel they are not alone and achieve a sense of peace with their life. Consider, for example, people's Christian belief, filtered through Catholic faith, that 'by way of Christ, God suffers with them'. Independent of such consolation from religious conviction or revelation is the potential for human suffering to act against the passive defencelessness and vulnerability of being human.

Suffering has this liberating power because it can even *enliven* those who suffer. Suffering has this paradoxical potential to vivify when it is viewed as a challenge to meet or accept within a quest narrative. As C.S. Lewis wrote, although 'pain hurts ... pain, below a certain level of intensity ... might even be rather liked'.[65] Pain and suffering can become integral to effortful progress toward happiness and flourishing. Indeed, people can be unhappy and happy at the same time. For example, from living with the muscular degenerative disease, Amyotrophic Lateral Sclerosis, the theologian–philosopher, Franz Rosenzweig exemplified, how, 'A condition into which one has slithered gradually, and consequently become used to, is not suffering but simply a condition ... that leaves room for joy and suffering like any other.'[66] The skills of happiness – as American psychologist, Martin Seligman noted in his 2004 TED talk – differ from those of relieving misery, and indeed the two states are related. Suffering helps persons to feel and celebrate the gift of life because, 'when we succeed in feeling nothing, we lose the only means we have of knowing what hurts, and why'.[67] Other reasons for the possibility of experiencing joy in the midst of suffering are the beauty of the world and the tendency of sick people to be mostly well and become awakened to the opportunity to care for others managing their suffering. For such reasons, finding the will to live on through a terrible condition and its impermanence can be lionizing and even revelled in, as Friedrich Nietzsche suggested, rather than necessarily produce (only) suffering, as suggested by Arthur Schopenhauer. Aware that society commonly exempts sick people from their usual responsibilities, patients may also happily crave the special attention that sickness can bring them.[68] Such benefits may depend on their willingness to participate in health care but act against alleviation of, or recovery from, sickness.

So, without diminishing the need of health care to relieve or minimize suffering, suffering can be less a problem to avoid at all costs than, as the philosopher Miguel de Unamuno opined, an essential part of the complexity of what it means to be human. To eliminate suffering is to extinguish life itself and, as the Buddha said, to desire what is beyond our grasp. So, without judging the appropriateness of individual patients' response to their state of health, I have suggested that compromising the primacy of patient welfare is the misnomer that patienthood connotes anguish, distress and debilitating suffering in the midst of sickness; some sick patients do not suffer. Other patients – sick and healthy – do suffer but their suffering does not necessarily make them passive and joyless or make their welfare paramount.

Similar patients are treated alike

De-emphasizing the need and ability to account for individual variability is a one-size-fits-all approach. Underwritten by population health care, which includes putting more epidemiology into personal health care, this commitment to standardize health care entails practices like implementing clinical guidelines and electronic health records to help clinicians reduce errors and ultimately save time and money. However, standardizing care provision can underestimate meaningful differences between the patients who present with the same problem or need. Critics of standardization argue that clinicians need to know and respond thoughtfully rather than mechanically to the nature and importance of the welfare and other moral interests of each patient and clinician. Evident in standardization, therefore, is a trend toward 'loss of the individual',[69] which promotes uniform clinical care that erodes patients' uniqueness and identity. Patients become 'faceless' as individual persons.

Patient-centred health care and, now, personalized medicine, both emphasize individualized care. However, patient-centred health care has been unable to resist the movement toward standardization, which in modern health care reflects at least two related sets of forces. The first of these takes a business focus, most notably in the United States, which commodifies health care and service relationships under a mass production model directed by general management in competitive and mixed markets. Characteristics of this volume-driven model include commercialization and, despite some decentralized authorities, a trend toward centralization and corporatization, for example through managed care enterprises. Pay-for-performance programmes, for example, draw on aggregate findings to incentivize clinician employees financially to adhere to clinical guidelines. The findings document performance against easily measurable professional standards that do not necessarily accommodate what individual patients want, especially when they become frail, disabled or live with serious chronic illness. To increase efficiency and accountability and cut rising costs, management structures have nevertheless weakened physicians' power to manage assorted patients differently. In contrast, pharmacists, for example, may welcome health policy changes such as reclassifying medicines from prescription to non-prescription, which increase their professional autonomy whilst also constraining it.

Second, in countries including the United Kingdom and New Zealand, a communitarian ethos undergirds policy requirements for health care practice to deliver population health care. This care is designed to contain costs; manage unintended variation in health care delivery; distribute health care resources fairly, when clinicians can confidently predict outcomes of interventions that are important to, and across, similar patients; and reduce health inequalities. The bright light shone from the political left by this health policy has cast a shadow over personal health care provision. This shadow anonymizes individual patients and creates a space for treating them largely the same rather than as individual persons. The source of the light here has been the convergence of clinical practice and public health, including the growth of a new scientific basis for clinical knowledge – epidemiology.

Increased epidemiology has been put into clinical practice through the development of evidence-based medicine, despite wide variation in implementing this practice model. On the basis of average results from clinical studies, and algorithmic rules, the normalizing gaze of evidence-based medicine risks sacrificing the individuality of clinicians and patients for the sake of health care interventions that, on balance, are marginally effective in the population. Any benefit to individual patients themselves depends on a 'probabilistic mode of reasoning that is systematically speculative'.[70] Proponents of evidence-based medicine rebut that their model emphasizes the clinical experience of the clinician in integrating research evidence with the clinical state and circumstances, and values and preferences, of individual patients.[71] They further note the methodological individualism of evidence-based medicine vis-à-vis upstream social influences on patient health outcomes, and the possibility of having both standardized care, such as systematic needs assessments, and responsive personalized care.[72] However, evidence-based medicine has never clearly explained how to use research evidence to individualize treatment decisions and fulfil its implicit promise to reduce health inequalities. Amid concern about the quality of much published research,[73] the exhortation to rationalize and standardize clinical practice opposes this need and tends to reproduce and reinforce social inequities. Especially in secondary health care, moreover, similarity is defined on the basis of an orientation to organ systems. Harry Callahan's photograph, *Eleanor 1947* gives visual presence to this reductionism. In a flattened sea of pale tonalities, this image of his wife gives selected focus to her eyes, detached from the whole person.

Therefore, standardized care is conducive to services that tend to be biomedical, specialized and fragmented in content, but potentially coordinated across user information networks even though population-level research cannot reliably predict what is best for each patient. Care that is bureaucratized and standardized also tends to weaken personal health care. Weakly responsive to context and uniqueness, standardized care resists understanding in situ and struggles to be receptive to distinctive patient risk profiles; to clinical presentations that include complex and common multimorbidity affecting each patient differently; and to values and preferences of individual patients. Its biomedical focus betrays private and public aspects of the lifeworlds of patients as situated persons. That, as Lucretius stated, 'One's man's meat is another man's poison', exposes a need to set boundaries on a Procrustean model of standardized care and explore alternatives; for example, for patients receiving total hip arthroplasty, a Swedish quasi-experiment found that compared with standardized care, involving them in decision-making reduced the mean length of the hospital stay.[74]

Patients remain unequal

While clinicians have treated similar patients alike, modern patients in particular are growing increasingly similar to clinicians,[75] undermining the need for patient-centred health care. Role convergence is taking place as education and communication technologies facilitate the production and diffusion of digital information to clinicians, from them to patients and between patients themselves. Unmanageable for clinicians, the sheer volume of this accessible health-related information on the Internet and World Wide Web is expanding the health literacy of patients. As part of a tendency for social processes to professionalize more and more people in the West, clinicians are gradually losing their monopoly over specialized health care knowledge in encounters with patients. Clinicians themselves reinforce this development by educating patients and aligning patients' values, capabilities and functions with their own to create more equal and democratic modes of clinician–patient interaction and decision-making. State-led reforms for health care reorganization, such as 'expert patient programmes' in the United Kingdom, have supported this social mobilization of patients, the changing nature of clinicianship and, on balance, converging role jurisdictions that amplify the unifying power of shared personhood. Yet, despite its commitment to shared decision-making and patient autonomy, patient-centred health care – premised on privileging patients by putting their welfare first – cannot ultimately accommodate these equalizing forces. Continuing asymmetries of power, especially between clinicians and non-modern patients, cannot salvage patient-centred health care. Nor can scepticism that even modern patients can always effectively process the value of information on the Internet and be experts on their health and health care.[76] As social roles continue to converge, they become increasingly incompatible with a model of health care centred on patients, a model promulgating a form of positive (or reverse) discrimination, even though positive discrimination is still discrimination.

3 Health has become a human 'commodified right'

The third set of issues undermining the primacy of patient welfare, and patient-centred health care, relates to the fundamental concept of a 'right to health' (care). In the United States, the PPACA offers protections known as the 'Patients' Bill of Rights', including health care coverage regardless of pre-existing medical conditions. However, a universal right to health is not exclusively a patient right. Protected by national constitutions and international agreements – most notably the International Covenant on Economic, Social and Cultural Rights ratified by most sovereign states, though not the United States – the right is a *human* right; an inherent right of every human being, not merely patients. Accordingly, clinicians, no less than patients, share the right independently of adopting the social role of patient. The moral justification for the right to health is unclear but over the past 70 years the modern notion of human rights has hinged on a determination to codify a new, universal standard of the dignity and equal moral worth of all human beings *as* human beings. Having the same moral worth by nature, human beings are entitled to the same moral rights. However, there is still no agreement today on the existence of human rights and their legitimacy and relevance in health care.

Support continues for Jeremy Bentham's influential critique, 200 years ago, of natural rights – and hence human rights – as 'nonsense upon stilts'. For Bentham, among others, rights are not metaphysical or theological. Rather they are social and political constructions within local communities. With respect therefore to the vague concept of a right to a decent 'minimum' level of health, one might argue that patient welfare comes first because the special risk or presence of illness among patients justifies their right to health ahead of other social groups. Patients satisfy the condition of the principle of utility expressed by Bentham, but not necessarily more so than the people who need health care to live a good life but choose not to adopt the role of patient to secure their right to it.

Moreover, why do states, if they really believe in primacy of patient welfare, restrict entitlement to the patients who can pay to access certain types of health care? And why have states needed to create a business case to incentivize professional behaviour among clinicians with weak intrinsic motivation to excel? These questions are important, not least because financing has challenged the ability of health systems to implement the right to health. Uncertain is the extent to which these systems are positively obligated to use their limited resources to realize basic claims implied by this right. The United States most conspicuously has treated health care as a commodity to which entitlement depends on how health markets, including health insurance markets, manage patients' ability and willingness to purchase and access health care. These 'markets serve themselves, not patients'[77] and typify the other health systems where clinicians charge for their services. Most of these systems mix publicly- and privately-financed health care services, in part commodifying health care. Thus, despite Michael Walzer's assertion that 'needed goods are not commodities',[78] health care has commonly become a 'commodified right'. Offered extrinsic incentives such as money, health care providers deliver health services as part of policy interventions like results-based financing. These interventions have been introduced because, despite social norms of professionalism, the intrinsic moral rewards such as pride and gratitude have lacked sufficient power to motivate clinicians to put patient welfare first.

4 Dehumanization cannot be morally functional

More than depersonalized, the clinical settings and practices performed every day have become increasingly 'dehumanized' in the sense of forfeiting qualities considered characteristically human. This dehumanization appears to lend support to the need for primacy of patient welfare. Implying an unmet need to put first the welfare of patients are what Omar Haque and Adam Waytz[79] describe as the 'non-functional' causes of dehumanization, namely: deindividuating practices, impaired patient agency and, despite role convergence, physician–patient dissimilarity. To reduce these problems, they prescribe individuation, agency reorientation and promoting similarity. However, these authors also identify 'functional' causes of dehumanization – mechanization, empathy reduction and moral disengagement – to meet professional demands inherent to effective health care delivery.[79,80] They suggest that, despite negative effects, some of these causes 'may be necessary for effective medical care when the dehumanization is transient and matched to direct clinical demands'. From their perspective therefore, health care can be functionally dehumanizing in order to put patient welfare first.

In contrast, I contend that the oxymoronic but now widely cited and rarely contested concept of functional dehumanization[80,81] raises serious ethical concerns. Undermining modern initiatives to revitalize humanism in health care, these concerns include reducing the patient – as a patient – to a mechanical object or automaton that lacks human qualities and does not therefore always require humanistic care. Dehumanizing the patient through acts that society misconstrues as defensible and even banal in their everydayness operates against the primacy of the welfare of the patient. Even if the patient experiences an expected, overall improvement in welfare, it seems wrong to use this end to license the clinician, in the name of benevolence, to perform humiliating and intimidating acts dispassionately; for patients may consent to the procedure rather than how it is performed. From this non-consequentialist position, dehumanization: is never morally appropriate, whatever its potential functionality in health care; is tantamount to a moral imposture that seduces clinicians into behaving badly; and dehumanizes the clinician. Even a clinical need to focus temporarily on a patient's body part (as when performing certain procedures) should aim to maximize the humanity of the whole person to whom the part belongs. Helping clinicians to meet this obligation is professional guidance on how to preserve dignity even during intimate clinical examinations.[82] One approach is clinician empathy.

As a dignity-enhancing value and practice of patient-centred health care, empathy informs understanding of the patient's perspective and can minimize patients' experience of isolation. However, when clinicians 'surface act' because they cannot immediately develop real emotion through 'deep acting',[83] their display of empathy is effectively deceptive and can be dehumanizing for both parties. Patients may feel unworthy of natural empathy and clinicians may experience negative emotions, such as guilt and shame, from not feeling and expressing empathy. Despite liberal arguments for feigning authentic emotions for the sake of equality and cooperation,[84-86] most patients want 'what is real'. They can frequently recognize inauthenticity and prefer not to waste their time receiving it. Hence, patient welfare is not put first by clinicians whom patient-centred health care has not required to reflect on their motives and be as genuinely caring as they can toward their patients.

Conclusion

All these developments cast doubt on the appropriateness and effectiveness of the model of patient-centred health care as a leading conceptualization of health care professionalism that requires clinicians to act not only in the best interests of individual patients but also to respect their autonomy and promote social justice. Requiring clinicians to balance these potentially competing interests is unreasonable. In turn, challenges to putting first the welfare of patients, while justly respecting the competence of their decisional capabilities, fracture clinicians' ability to care for patients across blurring social roles and populations. Clinicians cannot expect to perform this balancing act and receive trust from patients whose meaning and sense of entitlement to health care have been over-generalized without a clear, unifying relational space. A right to health does not depend on people adopting the role of patient. It is a human right to a social good that has become commodified in health systems lacking a clear commitment to the principle and feasibility of putting patient welfare first. Focusing on duty rather than motivation, moreover, patient-centred health care predisposes to insincerity, which provides a weak foundation for clinical care in which patients can feel confident.

References

1 Donabedian A. Evaluating the quality of medical care. *Milbank Memorial Fund Quarterly* 1966; 44: Supplement 166–206.

2 Institute of Medicine. *Crossing the Quality Chasm: A New Health System for the 21st Century*. Washington DC: National Academy Press; 2001.

3 Ackerknecht E. *Medicine at the Paris Hospital 1774–1848*. Baltimore: Johns Hopkins; 1967.

4 Armstrong D. The rise of surveillance medicine. *Sociology of Health and Illness* 1995; 17: 393–404.

5 Jewson ND. The disappearance of the sick-man from medical cosmology, 1770–1870. *Sociology* 1976; 10: 225–44.

6 Balint M. *The Doctor, His Patient, and the Illness*. London: Churchill Livingstone; 1957.

7 Balint E. The possibilities of patient-centred medicine. *Journal of the Royal College of General Practitioners* 1969; 17: 269–76.

8 Balint M, Ball DH, Hare ML. Training medical students in patient-centred medicine. *Comprehensive Psychiatry* 1969; 10: 249–58.

9 Huygen FJA. *Family Medicine; the Medical History of Families*. Nijmegen: Dekker en van der Vegt; 1978.

10 Levenstein J, McCracken E, McWhinney I, Stewart M, Brown JB. The patient-centred clinical method. 1. A model for the doctor-patient interaction in family medicine. *Family Practice* 1986; 3: 24–30.

11 Brown JB, Stewart M, McCracken E, McWhinney I, Levenstein J. The patient-centred clinical method. 2. Definition and application. *Family Practice* 1986; 3: 75–9.

12 Stewart M. Towards a global definition of patient centred care. *British Medical Journal* 2001; 322: 444–5.

13 Engel G. The need for a new medical model: a challenge for biomedicine. *Science* 1977; 196: 129–36.

14 Kleinman A, Eisenberg J, Good B. Culture, illness and care: clinical lessons from anthropologic and cross-cultural research. *Annals of Internal Medicine* 1978; 88: 251–8.

15 Charon R. *Narrative Medicine: Honoring the Stories of Illness*. New York: Oxford University Press; 2006.

16 Gerteis M, Edgman-Levitan S, Daley J, Delbanco TL, editors. *Through The Patient's Eyes*. San Francisco: Jossey-Bass; 1993.

17 Institute of Medicine. *Crossing the Quality Chasm: A New Health System for the 21st Century*. Washington DC: National Academy Press; 2001.

18 Picker Institute. *2011–12 Annual Report.* Camden, Maine: Picker Institute; 2011.

19 Fleurence R, Selby JV, Odom-Walker K, Hunt G, Meltzer D, Slutsky JR, Yancy C. How the Patient-Centered Outcomes Research Institute is engaging patients and others in shaping its research agenda. *Health Affairs* 2013; 32: 393–400.

20 Huerta TR, Sieck CJ, Hefner J, Johansen M, Wexler R, McAlearney AS. Patient-centred care plus medical home do not equal patient-centred medical home: why layering models of care may not lead to better outcomes. *OA Family Medicine* 2013; 1: 5.

21 Rathert C, Wyrwich MD, Boren SA. Patient-centered care and outcomes: a systematic review of the literature. *Medical Care Research and Review* 2013; 70: 351–79.

22 Friedberg MW, Schneider EC, Rosenthal MB, Volpp KG, Werner RM. Association between participation in a multipayer medical home intervention and changes in quality, utilization and costs of care. *Journal of the American Medical Association* 2014; 311: 815–25.

23 Duggan P, Geller G, Cooper L, Beach M. The moral nature of patient-centeredness: is it 'just the right thing to do'? *Patient Education and Counseling* 2006; 62: 271–6.

24 Beauchamp T, Childress JF. *Principles of Biomedical Ethics.* First edition. Oxford: Oxford University Press; 1979.

25 ABIM Foundation, ACP-ASIM Foundation, European Federation of Internal Medicine. Medical professionalism in the new millennium: a physician charter. *Annals of Internal Medicine* 2002; 136: 243–6.

26 Cassel C, Hood V, Bauer W. A physician charter: the 10th anniversary. *Annals of Internal Medicine* 2012; 157: 290–1.

27 Polder J, Jochemsen H. Professional autonomy in the health care system. *Theoretical Medicine and Bioethics* 2000; 21: 477–91.

28 Zaner, R. Physicians and patients in relation: clinical interpretation and dialogues of trust. In: Khushf, G, editor. *Handbook of Bioethics. Taking Stock of the Field from a Philosophical Perspective.* Dordrecht: Kluwer 2004; pp. 223–50.

29 NHS England. Putting patients first. The NHS England business plan for 2013/14–2015/16. Redditch: NHS England; 2013.

30 Wendler D. Are physicians obligated always to act in the patient's best interests? *Journal of Medical Ethics* 2010; 36: 66–70.

31 Jotkowitz A, Glick S. The physician charter on medical professionalism: a Jewish ethical perspective. *Journal of Medical Ethics* 2005; 31: 404–5.

32 Gillon R. 'The patient's interests always come first'? Doctors and society. *British Medical Journal* 1986; 292: 398–400.

33 Sox H. Editorial. Medical professionalism in the new millennium: a physician charter. *Annals of Internal Medicine* 2002; 136: 243.

34 Cohen JJ, Cruess S, Davidson C. Alliance between society and medicine. The public's stake in medical professionalism. *Journal of the American Medical Association* 2007; 298: 670–3.

35 Delbanco T, Berwick D, Boufford JI, Edgman-Levitan S, Ollenschlager G, Plamping D, Rockefeller R. Healthcare in a land called PeoplePower: nothing about me without me. *Health Expectations* 2001; 4: 144–50.

36 Oshana M. How much should we value autonomy? In: Paul EF, Miller FDJ, Paul J, editors. *Autonomy.* Cambridge: Cambridge University Press 2003; pp. 99–126.

37 Berwick D. What 'patient-centered' should mean: confessions of an extremist. *Health Affairs* 2009; 28: w555–w565.

38 McNutt R. Shared decision-making: optional v mandatory autonomy of patients.

Family medicine should support the optional autonomy of patients in decision-making: the negative argument. In: Buetow S, Kenealy T, editors. *Ideological Debates in Family Medicine.* New York: Nova Science Publishers Inc 2007; pp. 251–9.

39 Minami C, Yang A, Szmuilowicz E. Negotiating the tensions in patient-centered care. *Journal of the American Medical Association* 2015; 314: 1167–8.

40 Veatch R. Character formation in professional education: a word of caution. In: Kenny N, Shelton W, editors. *Lost Virtue (Advances in Bioethics, Volume 10).* Bingley: Emerald Group Publishing 2006; pp. 29–45.

41 Beauchamp TL, Childress JF. *Principles of Biomedical Ethics.* Sixth edition. Oxford: Oxford University Press; 2009.

42 Brudney D, Lantos J. Agency and authenticity: which value grounds patient choice? *Theoretical Medicine and Bioethics* 2011; 32: 217–27.

43 O'Neill O. *Autonomy and Trust in Bioethics.* Cambridge: Cambridge University Press; 2005.

44 Miles SH. *The Hippocratic Oath and the Ethics of Medicine.* Oxford: Oxford University Press; 2004.

45 Love C. Family group conferencing. Cultural origins, sharing, and appropriation – a Maori reflection. In: Burford G, Hudson J, editors. *Family Group Conferencing. New Directions in Community-Centered Child and Family Practice.* Third edition. Piscataway, New Jersey: Transaction 2009; pp. 15–30.

46 White K. *Healing the Schism: Epidemiology, Medicine and the Public's Health.* New York: Springer-Verlag; 1991.

47 World Health Organization. *Alma-Ata Declaration on Primary Health Care.* Geneva: WHO; 1978.

48 Kindig D, Stoddart G. What is population health? *American Journal of Public Health* 2003; 93: 380–3.

49 Rose G. *The Strategy of Preventive Medicine.* Oxford: Oxford University Press; 1992.

50 Angell M. The doctor as double agent. *Kennedy Institute of Ethics Journal* 1993; 3: 279–86.

51 Swick H, Bryan C, Longo L. Beyond the Physician Charter: reflections on medical professionalism. *Perspectives in Biology and Medicine* 2006; 49: 263–75.

52 Pendleton D, King J. Values and leadership. *British Medical Journal* 2002; 325: 1352–5.

53 Baudrillard J. *The Transparency of Evil.* London: Verso; 2009.

54 Marinker M. Why make people patients? *Journal of Medical Ethics* 1975; I: 81–4.

55 Morris D. Illness and health in the postmodern age. *Advances in Mind-Body Medicine* 1998; 14: 237–51.

56 Heath I. Family medicine should focus on the 'sick': affirmative position. In: Buetow S, Kenealy T, editors. *Ideological Debates in Family Medicine.* New York: Nova Biomedical Books 2007; pp. 73–81.

57 Cholesterol Treatment Trialists' (CTT) Collaborators, Mihaylova B, Emberson J, Blackwell L, Keech A, Simes J, Barnes EH, Voysey M, Gray A, Collins R, Baigent C. The effects of lowering LDL cholesterol with statin therapy in people at low risk of vascular disease: meta-analysis of individual data from 27 randomised trials. *Lancet* 2012; 380(9841): 581–90. doi:http://dx.doi.org/10.1016/S0140-6736(12)60367-5.

58 Ebrahim S, Casas JP. Statins for all by the age of 50 years? *Lancet* 2012; 380(9841): 545–7.

59 Stone NJ, Robinson JG, Lichtenstein AH, Bairey Merz CN, Blum CB, Eckel RH, Goldberg AC, Gordon D, Levy D, Lloyd-Jones DM, McBride P, Schwartz JS, Shero

ST, Smith SC Jr, Watson K, Wilson PW. 2013 ACC/AHA guideline on the treatment of blood cholesterol to reduce atherosclerotic cardiovascular risk in adults: a report of the American College of Cardiology/American Heart Association Task Force on Practice Guidelines. *Journal of the American College of Cardiology* 2014; 63(25 Pt B): 2889–934.

60 Steiner-Grossman P. *The New People, Not Patients: A Source Book for Living with Inflammatory Bowel Disease.* New York: Crohns and Colitis Foundation of America; 1997.

61 Pellegrino ED. Medical ethics in an era of bioethics: resetting the medical profession's compass. *Theoretical Medicine and Bioethics* 2012; 33: 21–4.

62 Frankl V. *Man's Search for Meaning: An Introduction to Logotherapy.* Boston: Beacon Press; 1963.

63 Lebacqzk K. The virtuous patient. In: Shelp E, editor. *Virtue and Medicine.* Dordrecht: Kluwer Academic Publishers 1985; pp. 275–88.

64 May R. *The Meaning of Anxiety.* New York: WW Norton and Company; 1977.

65 Lewis CS. *The Problem of Pain.* London: Collins; 1940.

66 Glatzer NN. *Franz Rosenzweig: His Life and Thought.* Indianapolis: Hackett Publishing; 1998.

67 Grosz S. *The Examined Life. How we Lose and Find Ourselves.* London: Vintage; 2014.

68 Williams W. Behavioural anomalies in patients and doctors. II Secondary gain, or the advantages of being 'sick'. In: Ellard J, editor. *Psychiatry for the Non-Psychiatrist.* Sydney: Geigy Pharmaceuticals 1978; pp. 167–72.

69 Heath I. Overdiagnosis: when good intentions meet vested interests. *British Medical Journal* 2013; 346: f6361.

70 Fox R. Toward an ethics of iatrogenesis. In: Lafleur W, Böhme H, Shimazono S, editors. *Dark Medicine. Rationalizing Unethical Medical Research.* Bloomington: Indiana University Press 2007; pp. 149–64.

71 Haynes R, Devereaux P, Guyatt G. Clinical expertise in the era of evidence-based medicine and patient choice. *ACP Journal Club* 2002; 136: A11–14.

72 Hynes SM. Is it possible to have both standardised and person-centred care? *International Journal of Geriatric Psychiatry* 2015; 30: 431–2.

73 Ioannidis J. Why most published research findings are false. *PLoS Medicine* 2005; 2: e124.

74 Olsson L-E, Karlsson J, Berg J, Kärrholm J, Hansson E. Person-centred care compared with standardized care for patients undergoing total hip arthroplasty – a quasi-experimental study. *Journal of Orthopaedic Surgery and Research* 2014; 9: 95.

75 Buetow S, Jutel A, Hoare K. Shrinking social space in the doctor-modern patient relationship: a review of forces for, and implications of, role convergence. *Patient Education and Counseling* 2009; 74: 97–103.

76 Prior L. Belief, knowledge and expertise: the emergence of the lay expert in medical sociology. *Sociology of Health Illness* 2003; 25: 41–57.

77 Geyman J. Family medicine should emphasize the provision of health care as a social good: affirmative position. In: Buetow S, Kenealy T, editors. *Ideological Debates in Family Medicine.* New York: Nova Science 2007; pp. 221–8.

78 Walzer M. *Spheres of Justice.* New York: Basic Books; 1983.

79 Haque O, Waytz A. Dehumanization in medicine: causes, solutions, and functions. *Perspectives on Psychological Science* 2012; 7: 176–86.

80 Leyens J. Humanity forever in medical dehumanization. In: Bain P, Vaes J, Leyes J, editors. *Humanness and Dehumanization.* New York: Psychology Press 2014; pp. 167–85.

81 Haslam N, Loughnan S. Dehumanization and infrahumanization. *Annual Review of Psychology* 2014; 65: 399–423.

82 General Medical Council. Intimate examinations and chaperones. 2013; Available at: www.gmc-uk.org/guidance/ethical_guidance/21168.asp. Accessed 6 March 2015.

83 Larson E, Yao X. Clinical empathy as emotional labor in the patient-physician relationship. *Journal of the American Medical Association* 2005; 293: 1100–6.

84 Waskul DW. The importance of insincerity and inauthenticity for self and society: why honesty is not the best policy. In: Vannini P, Williams P, editors. *Authenticity in Culture, Self, and Society.* Farnham, Surrey: Ashgate Publishing 2009; pp. 51–64.

85 de Mandeville B. *The Fable of the Bees.* Printed for J. Tonson: London; 1724.

86 Kang J. Uses of insincerity. *Law and Literature* 2003; 15: 371–93.

3 Patient self-care

Introduction

Filling the frame of Otto Umbehr's (Umbo's) photographic *Portrait of Ruth Landshoff (The Hat)* is the borderless close-up of a young German actress. Her half-turned movement out of the frame helps to shield her from the bright light of the public gaze. So too do the shadow draped by the hat above her eyes and the bleached authenticity washing the lower half of her face. At the same time, this cosmetically manufactured appearance – including dark lipstick, slightly open mouth and wide brimmed, latticed hat – coyly solicits approval from the public light. This image gives symbolic form to the active but exposed and vulnerable role played by many patients today across private–public spaces on the stage of modern health care. The quasi-public light of this care makes increasingly visible how patients act. Believing that those who see them tend to judge them – for example on their physical appearance – these patients may put on their best face to give at least a picture of the health of their socialized body and life. Prompted also to look for things wrong inside themselves, they may use this picture to mask anxiety about their inner health[1,2] and reinforce their self-conscious need to become increasingly risk-conscious and health abiding. This behaviour reflects and feeds apprehension of a 'dark side' of healthy self-care as a regulative ideal of 'good citizens' in late modern society.[3]

Whether the self-care scripted by patient-centred health care, and blurring with care from clinicians, ameliorates patients' welfare can be unclear from a health system perspective. At least for long-term illness, self-care for health often produces modest benefits in randomized controlled trials.[4,5] In this context patient-centred health care has battled to demonstrate the efficacy of its construction of healthy self-care. At the same time it has struggled to acknowledge as self-care the myriad choices that patients actually make to care for themselves on their own terms, for some patients self-care differently than society expects for their health. They seek to care for their welfare in personally meaningful ways that patient-centred health care illuminates but might not recognize as self-care. For example, patients may self-care in ways independent of even a semblance of health. To these patients, self-care need not promote health despite most of the many definitions of self-care emphasizing this particular focus.[6]

From this perspective I define patient self-care as care actively helping patients to self-realize their capabilities to flourish and live well in ways faithful to deep, defensible values they may come to recognize in themselves. This concern for authenticity as a dimension of autonomy goes beyond patient-centred health care's focus on autonomy in terms of agency for health care. Nevertheless an unmet need exists to ensure patients can cultivate and exercise good character in order to bridge different positions on self-care by addressing interests relevant to themselves and their clinician.[7]

This chapter will address these complex issues. After looking at how patient self-care has developed over time as a potential resource, it will discuss the scope of the meaning of the patient self and the importance, to patient-centred health care, of health for self-care in the general population. After considering the diverse ways in which patients seek to self-care, the chapter will consider patients' capabilities and responsibilities for self-care within health care, including implications for patient autonomy. Despite suggesting sympathetically that patients choose to self-care in ways that go beyond health, I temper my liberalism by noting that self-care cannot be whatever patients want to make it. Self-care requires that patients strive to know and show fidelity to their moral values, interests and capabilities to live well within a life project of virtue-cultivation in their own particular circumstances.

Development of self-care

Patient self-care is not a new phenomenon. Everyday health care has always depended on patients caring for themselves and each other. Patients have mostly self-cared in private spaces, such as households and family settings, as well as in workplaces and local communities.[8] Many self-care tasks of patients in these settings have routinely fallen to women. Yet health systems have commonly failed to acknowledge the importance of these devotional, lay practices[9] – especially with the growth of institutionalized health care in the nineteenth century. The advent of hospital medicine and then laboratory medicine transformed medicine from a person-oriented cosmology toward an object-oriented one,[10] clearly separating formal health care from informal health care including self-care. Over about the last half-century, this distinction has weakened. Lay participation has grown in social life and health care as a common good. Within new relational forms of mixed care, expansion of self-care has split the burden of health care delivery to respect patient autonomy – including patient choice and participation – manage rising financial costs, and try to improve patient health outcomes. With the shift toward chronic illness management, and the rise of consumerism and patient-centred health care, many patients have accepted this role to share control over their health. Within converging spaces of domestic and work life, they have co-produced novel geographies of self-care.

Moving beyond the 'looked after' and compliant sick patient idealized by Talcott Parsons[11] in the 1950s, these new social arrangements have, despite some dissent, given social and public solidarity to self-care as a social movement.

This movement has deterritorialized and refashioned self-care as a collective activity in which patients have increased health consciousness, autonomy and independence. Patient demand for, and expectations of, self-care have grown in response – spurred by ideologies that in the 1960s and 1970s promoted universal entitlement to health care; in the 1980s and 1990s supported a shift toward market mechanisms; and in subsequent years have enhanced access to, and support for, increasing self-management and personalized self-service. These recent developments have been enabled by integrating markets, for example through public policies for legally reclassifying or switching medicines from prescription only to non-prescription sale, and from mobilizing communities through forces such as education and new and emergent health technologies.

In *The Patient Will See You Now*, for example, Eric Topol[12] envisions a future in which patients perform many functions of today's clinicians. Making possible this expanded self-care are developments in digital media information and communication technologies. A growing range of mobile apps and other devices enables patients to access online – anywhere, anytime – interactive and personalized websites, coaching software, support networks, social media platforms and other interconnected electronic systems. Such technologies are equipping patients with the knowledge, skills, motivation and other resources to help perform tasks like diagnostic testing and monitoring. In ageing populations, such technology-mediated change in self-care promises to help manage risks and the growth in demand for health care of long-term illness, and to promote health in the community.

While reducing or, more accurately, shifting and sharing the financial costs of health care, these developments are weakening limitations of institutional care, including the ability of clinicians to monitor and oversee daily living, minor ailments and chronic conditions from the perspective of patients. Their lay perspective is especially important when their priorities differ from those of clinicians. Among people with Parkinson's disease, for example, care management of daily burdens to maintain mood and quality of life can be more important than the severity of their neurodegenerative disorder and the effectiveness of drug treatments.[13] They and clinicians can bridge their interests through active participation in partnerships for self-care, shared decision-making and concordance. Many patients today want to play such a full and informed role in their self-care. They construct self-care as a resource that, to live well, they may focus on to support their own health within modern societies that have expanded the meaning of self-care beyond constructs of a personal self.

Self-sacrifice

A difficulty with self-care – exacerbated rather than lessened by patient-centred health care – is the uncertain meaning of selfhood. Scholars have long debated whether selfhood and personal identity exist beyond experience, and change over time. However, by viewing different perspectives as conversational partners rather than opposing viewpoints, I recognize the self as potentially essential *and* simultaneously emergent. The latter approach characterizes George Herbert Mead's theory of the social self, according to which the self combines two sides that develop over time through social interactions. The 'I' is how one personally identifies in response to the socialized self of 'me'.

Through patient-centred health care's commitment to preventive care and health promotion, the 'me' has expanded to include the population. The patient – not only the clinician – is expected now to balance competing allegiances as a 'double agent', advocating for their own lay interests but also helping to manage scarce public resources for the collective good. Indeed, society and clinicians exercise social control by imbuing feelings of personal responsibility in patients to walk an even thinner tightrope. Patients may understand and value the importance of civic-mindedness and community care but what they tend not to understand is the expectation on them to subordinate their autonomy and welfare to the population health. Subordination takes place through self-care activities that tend directly to benefit others more than themselves, and carry personal risks. Such activities include vaccinating individuals at low risk of rare or rarely serious diseases to achieve herd immunity. Does this public expectation take self-care too far? Rather than support personal self-care, it risks immolating the patient on the altar of social justice amid lack of transparency – conditions that weaken patients' most important relationship: their relationship with themselves, on which care of other persons depends. For this reason, Aristotle encouraged people to love themselves as their best friend. And the rhetorical question insightfully posed by the Rabbi, Hillel the Elder elucidates why: 'If I am not for myself, who will be for me? But if I am only for myself, who am I? If not now, when?'

Healthism

Initiatives to develop a culture of health, including a social expectation to care for the 'common self' or population, further socialize and enculturate patients – in particular the proto-professionalized middle classes. Patients are led to view self-care in terms of privileging healthy living over other values to support human functioning and welfare and make the most of life's opportunities. Social strategies to support healthy behaviour include serial, not always well-coordinated reminders from clinics and clinicians to participate in surveillance programmes such as breast screening, and media awareness campaigns for healthy eating and safe sex. Problems arise when such appeals feel intimidating.

Fear appeals, for example, can illustrate a culture of potentially 'coercive healthism'.[14] Clinicians can be incentivized to cooperate, ostensibly for patients' own good, and through the lure of receiving payments to include very sick patients in the denominators of performance metrics like cancer screening. Amid concepts like 'preventionitis' and the 'health police',[15] this culture can cast patients adrift and drown their sense of autonomy. Loss of personal freedom persists for the sake of health even though much of health care – including contraception, fertility treatments, sports medicine and plastic surgery – has less to do with health than with healing or finding happiness and meaning in life. Despite this fact, self-care exclusively for health can suffocate rather than rescue patients. Vigilance in supporting uptake targets for cancer screening, for example, can save lives but also create patients who, ill-informed about screening risks, sink needlessly into the depths of worry about having medical conditions whose malignant potential may be unpredictable, and which they might be better off not knowing about and not having treated. In the absence of a personalized balancing of risks and benefits of individual forms of self-care, these shadows – real and imagined like those depicted in William Rimmer's painting, *Flight and Pursuit* – can inappropriately frighten people into accepting unsafe health care to try to escape possible danger from disease they might not be able to avoid.

The pervasiveness of these problems cannot be easily overestimated. Consider people's constant, often media-driven fear that danger threatens their health in every corner of daily life. Mocking the occasional remonstrations that patients are not 'afraid enough'[16] is a pernicious 'epidemic of apprehension'.[17] It deters patients from entertaining risky lifestyle behaviour that might enrich their life; impels them to try to self-care in ways that lack clear personal benefit, while exposing them to potential harms; and sensitizes and agitates them to notice, report and seek help for an expanding number of real and imagined symptoms and imperfections.[18] Paradoxically, however, other patients may avoid or delay seeking clinical care for their concerns if they fear being asked – or given unsolicited advice – about unrelated health issues. This milieu for preventative care and health promotion acts against self-care. For example, consider personal and public health messages that depict being overweight, and not merely obese, as a disease rather than a choice or biological adaptation, and prompt self-care via intentional weight loss through dieting and other lifestyle behaviour change.

A recent viewpoint in the *Journal of the American Medical Association* mistakenly assumes that patient health incentives for weight loss produce 'health and financial benefits without any risks'.[19] The viewpoint was suggesting that, compared with weight loss, incentivized breast screening better exemplifies the ethical need to balance potential benefits and harms. Yet even weight loss programmes are not necessarily conducive to self-care. They provoke patients to self-scrutinize their weight, and fear being, or becoming, overweight or obese even though 'Not all patients classified as being overweight or having grade 1 obesity, particularly those with chronic diseases, can be assumed to require weight loss treatment.'[20] This conclusion accompanies an editorial on a recent systematic review and meta-analysis[21] reporting lower mortality among people who are overweight than normal weight, as defined by the Body Mass Index alone. As an imperfect predictor of metabolic risk, this index has long been known to be inadequate as a health risk phenotype, taking no account of factors like fat distribution, nutritional status or cardiorespiratory fitness. Health concerns about overweight have continued nevertheless to be oversimplified, unhelpfully encouraging people to appraise themselves on the basis of how they look against contemporary idealized standards and to feel responsible for, and guilty about, their deviations from these standards. Women in particular face pressure from weight loss promoters with often questionable motives to conform to an elusive and stereotyped 'beauty myth'. This pressure can lead to unhealthy weight cycling and eating disorders, among other things.

The common-sense model of self-regulation of health and illness[22] assumes that people naturally self-regulate their health-related behaviour to avoid or minimize illness and its adverse effects. However, healthism has contributed to a sense of personal self so fragile that its care can commonly require constant support from others. In this environment many patients increasingly seek such support from connectivity across digital media, which creates for patients its own anxieties around loss of independence, depletion of time for reflection, and periods of disconnection from virtual relationships in which machines mediate intimacy. Other anxieties include loss of privacy, through possible surveillance of self-care, by patients who seek protection in the bubble of their ego amid the erosion in society of the personal self and healthy relationships. Adding to the need for self-care, this quest produces a vicious circle by increasing connectivity online. Moreover, while clinicians promote health care, they may inappropriately respect patient choices unfaithful to deep values of the patient.

Turning healthism on its head, clinicians can condone – even promote – patients' inauthentic behaviour, as when patients claim to want to be healthy but refuse, for example, to try to stop unhealthy behaviour like problem gambling or smoking after life-saving surgery that their smoking has contributed to or has complicated. If these patients need the surgery to be healthy enough to restart smoking, then some clinical intervention is needed. Similarly, many hospitals condone smoking outside them by gowned patients attached to drips. In 2013 in the United Kingdom, a National Institute for Clinical Excellence proposal to end this practice was widely criticized as inhumane.[23] Yet the problem is not inhumanity toward patients under stress but giving them moral licence to make whatever choices they legally want, even when these choices are inauthentic and lack moral integrity.

Forms of self-care

Expanding the range of vision of patient-centred health care, patients choose to self-care in ways that go beyond participation in conventional activities to achieve, maintain or restore health. To discuss this observation I want to depict, zoomorphically, six groups of patients respectively as sheep, giraffes, ants, dolphins, peacocks and eagles. These groups fit the abstract model of 'ideal types' that approximates the reality of how some patients behave but, without prescribing how they ought to act, accentuates and synthesizes some of their values, beliefs and conduct. Recognizing that patients may move between and even straddle ideal types, which are less distinct than they may appear, I will examine each group in relation to patient-centred health care. The groups discussed are not exhaustive. However, in illustrating how patient-centred health care suits sheep better than the other creatures, they expose a need for a new care model.

This model would accommodate diverse forms of self-care that patients adopt in good faith to live well and achieve quality of life within a tenable moral matrix.

Sheep

Sheep are the patients most readily associated with self-care, as promoted by patient-centred health care. Instinctively apprehensive of threats to their health, they seek protection within the comfort of the flock, pastorally guided by the clinician as a shepherd delivering population health care. Redolent of the shepherd–flock motif in literary discourse, these patients learn to recognize, trust and follow where their clinician is taking them without critical questioning and much understanding. As social beings whose nature is to please, sheep-like patients are content to be led – among incurious others – to the high ground of perceived safety. In following this path they risk sacrificing themselves for the sake of the group. If all patients were sheep, patient-centred health care would suffice to meet the collective health need of patients for self-care. However, this hypothetical is no endorsement of sheepish behaviour or patient-centred health care because, 'to be fully virtuous, it is not enough to act correctly by following tradition, for instance, or by unreflectively taking someone else's lead'.[24] That said, many patients demonstrate different traits of character represented symbolically by other creatures.

Giraffes

Giraffes resemble sheep in having a strong sense of self-protection within their communities. However, giraffes recognize the value but also the limitations of mainstream, reductionist health sciences as well as heterodox, holistic traditions. Giraffes respect the latter practices for their capacity to nurture the healing power of nature. To negotiate the range distinction between what is 'natural' rather than 'artificial', giraffes *integrate* conventional health care and evidence-informed, complementary self-care approaches. Reticulating these channels of interest and protection allows giraffes to optimize self-healing and pragmatically blend with their different habitats, even though giraffes also stick their neck out. They raise their head above the parapet of allopathic patient-centred medicine to make balanced and creative self-care choices. With gentle independence and courage, these choices connect giraffes' inner world to their external environment where they can live fully, simply and in good faith. Understanding that perfect health is an illusion and that life is unpredictable, giraffes may further exercise virtues such as purity and temperance without asceticism. Rather than act like sheep, for example, by simply following advice to avoid drinking alcohol, the giraffes (who may perceive alcohol as natural) choose to minimize its consumption, or even to drink a little customarily to lower their total risk of death.[25] Commitment devices, such as buying alcohol in small quantities, may be used to help. Other times, giraffes may opt out of self-care interventions, like particular vaccinations and screening tests for conditions such as prostate cancer[26] and breast cancer,[27] because public health programmes have exaggerated their benefits and downplayed their risks. Giraffes' distinctiveness lessens however as their numbers swell upon putting themselves at the centre of public attention in modern communities whose progressive individualism promotes tolerance of, and even attraction to, integration.

Ants

Ants self-care by cooperating with, and caring for, others, including clinicians as well as themselves. While sheep tend, non-reflectively, to follow the flock, ants are thoughtful, proactive and purposeful team players. Like giraffes, they practise preventive health care in prudent good faith. But ants go further; they self-care by interacting patiently and in harmony for the *common good* – the community as a whole – by serving, and in a sense 'being', their colonies unified by shared health concerns. From this mindset of solidarity with others in need, they accept and share responsibility for doing what they can themselves, constitutionally as the community, by exhibiting socially responsible self-care behaviour. These patients are the kind who, for the good of society, accept vaccinations currently conferring negligible personal benefits; refrain from smoking in public spaces; use antibiotics prudently to reduce antibiotic resistance in communities; and participate in clinical trials. In so doing, they act less as patients than as citizens – as persons of virtue. 'The ants ...' wrote Peter Kropotkin, 'have renounced the "Hobbesian war" and they are the better for it.'[28] Note that their civic virtue goes beyond patient-centred personal health care, which is quiet on how, as mentioned in the Book of Proverbs (30:25), virtue makes ants into people who behave like ants; just as, in Ovid's *Metamorphoses*, in answer to his son's prayers for company on the island of Aegina, Zeus changed a colony of ants into human beings who, 'true to their origin ... still have their customary talents'.[29]

Dolphins

Dolphins exemplify the human drive to experience *pleasure*. The English moral philosopher, Bernard Williams[30] observed that, 'many people are horrible because they are unhappy'. Dolphin-like patients seek happiness through enjoying themselves playfully with others. Here, self-care includes socially liberal attitudes and behaviour, for example toward alcohol and sex. Two dolphin pods appear salient. The first seeks pleasure which its members expect to exceed their risk of experiencing pain or suffering (the 'pleasure principle'). Motivating the second pod is the expected *jouissance* of pleasure *regardless* – or, as exemplified by gambling, even *because* – of the risks. As a potentially exciting way to resist stifling cultural norms, the risks associated with pleasure-seeking may motivate rather than deter unhealthy self-care behaviour (reactance theory[31]) despite the fact that, in general, these dolphins would rather be healthy than unhealthy. Different cognitive states characterize the two pods.

Acting from reason: The first pod, in particular, may believe, on the basis of strong reasons, that pleasure-seeking is subjectively and defensibly rational – though their thinking may be objectively mistaken[32] – since gains from unhealthy pleasure outweigh empirical risks. This 'cognitivist theory of action' may also apply to the second pod, for which *jouissance* is subjectively rational. Cognisant that 'low risk' or 'safe' behaviour is ultimately subjective and uncertain, this pod reasons that pleasure is desirable for its own sake and questions privileging health over other, pleasurable aspects of daily life. For example, as Samuel Taylor Coleridge reasoned in his song, *Drinking Versus Thinking*, 'Let's live while we are able.' Coleridge and other mystics constructed lifestyle activities like drinking as subjectively rational sources of creative and subversive energy. Drug ingestion freed them from felt incompleteness and, while facilitating sociality, from enslavement to social conformity. More than a social lubricant for self-expression, alcohol and opiates opened doors to transcendental experience of an authentic life. In such circumstances, as the Situationist, Raoul Vaneigem clarified, 'The eruption of lived pleasure is such that in losing myself I find myself; forgetting that I exist I realize myself.'[33] These dolphins further self-care when, with an open mind, they trust others fully to accept and endorse them in this state, not merely for who they are but also *despite* who they are. Others' acceptance of these dolphins' darker side, including even defiling behaviour that lays bare unrespectable impulses, replaces fear and shame and satisfies an otherwise repressed need for intimacy. In contrast, a second state of cognition characterizes self-care by the second dolphin pod.

Acting against reason: From hunger for *jouissance* these dolphins do not care whether their unhealthy lifestyle choices debase them. They act consciously not from subjective rationality but against their own reasoning. Referred to by the French philosopher and historian, Michel Foucault as having the condition of *stultitia* – described much earlier by the Roman Stoic philosopher and statesman, Seneca – they recognize the rationality of living healthily, for example because health facilitates happiness. Stultified nevertheless by their passions within, and by desires ignited from the outside world, they are unwilling or unable to adhere to reason and minimize risks to their health by restricting themselves to experience of healthy pleasure. Stigmatizing themselves for the madness of behaving, in the moment, contrary to their own reasoning,[34] they persist in unhealthy, pleasure-seeking behaviour, in part because it is a (maladaptive) form of self-care. Wrestling with feelings like guilt, their self-care is a form of submission marked by a vicious circle between self-pleasure and self-blame – or *ressentiment* – that gives meaning to suffering they neurotically may also seek out.

Self-care? Dolphins with *stultitia* are open to changing self-care behaviour through patient-centred health care. In contrast, those acting subjectively rationally value patient-centred health care's commitment to respect their values and preferences but discern and reject this model's value premise that patients ought to follow norms of healthy living to help prevent and manage disease. Characterizing sociopolitically the complex relationship between morality and health, these norms tend to regulate lifestyle behaviour, explicitly or implicitly. For example, in implicitly dispensing moral prescriptions for healthy living, health promotion discourse is quiet on how responsible usage of pornography may safely help adults to explore and express their sexuality – despite saturation of popular culture with sexual imagery and common demand for, and patronage of, pornography. It is as if the clinician has one eye open and one eye closed – as well as being closed-mouthed, as observed in Pablo Picasso's preparatory sketch, *The Head of the Medical Student*. The same characterization applies to the patient who recognizes no need to focus attention on health goals, find common ground or share decision-making with the clinician about their lifestyle behaviour. These patients want to stay faithful in their self-care to their moral values and freedoms, so they resist health care committed to changing health-compromising or morally uncertain behaviour that restricts pleasure.

Smoking provokes an even more challenging test of the adequacy of patient-centred health care as a model describing how some dolphins seek to self-care. This model rejects as self-care the unhealthy pleasure experienced by these smokers, whether they act on the basis of their reasoning or against their own reasoning. Generally aware of the serious health risks of smoking, even subjectively rational dolphins may reason that satisfying benefits from smoking exceed the health risks. These risks may appear to lie in the deep future or these smokers may reason that they are likely in their social milieu to die young anyway; and, from personal experience, they feel better when they smoke, or else they would not smoke. Smoking gives them sensory pleasure, reduces their stress and anxiety levels and – by providing an opportunity for creative pause from, and reflection on, life – helps them cope with daily problems and function at work, in social situations, or both. Smoking frees them from repressive self-denial of pleasure that requires subordinating themselves to healthy living. For these smokers, these reasoned benefits equate to living well and self-care. They construct smoking, at least when they begin this practice, as a liberating habit that enables them to be faithful to human needs, rather than a problem of dependence or addiction. Hence they eschew health care whose purpose is to help them avoid smoking-related disease. In this context a challenge for health care – de-emphasized by patient-centred health care – is to ensure the values, beliefs and agency of patients are not merely fully informed but also are coherent and consistent with their moral sense of who they are. Only then can the authenticity of personal lifestyle choices make these choices truly autonomous and respectable.

Peacocks

Peacocks self-care by using health care for purposes over and above health. To visibly improve their form or functioning beyond their normal, healthy state, they access continuing advances in enhancement biotechnologies such as aesthetic medicine and psychopharmaceuticals. Even though they might not lack health, their sense of self-worth may hinge on them using the technologies to (re)create themselves outwardly and inwardly; display with pride the person they want to become; dispose others to infer their good character from their outer appearance; and feel special. Often underlying their apparent egocentrism is fragile self-esteem and vulnerability.[35] Consciously or not, enhancement can answer their cry for freedom, which overlaps with my discussion of what motivates dolphins. Yet it can be difficult to know whether or when bioenhancement aims to be liberating and therapeutic; and also unclear is patient-centred health care's ability to accommodate these nuances.

Critical of human enhancements, so-called anti-meliorists question whether the bioenhancements are self-caring, whatever their motivation. They point out that the enhancements are artificial, medicalize life; divert scarce health care resources from relief of sick patients; widen social inequalities and can be vainfully self-perpetuating.[36] Yet if patients are to be free to define self-care in a personally meaningful manner, they need to be able to make their own moral choices on how to act on this self-definition. For example, consider cosmetic breast augmentation for, and requiring, self-care. This procedure reinforces sexist stereotypes about how women need to appear in order to be considered attractive in western patriarchal culture – and has been associated with increased personal health risks including suicide.[37] Nevertheless, many women make an informed choice to undergo this surgical procedure to help them achieve their life goals and care for themselves in a world already deeply unnatural. Breast augmentation and its growing normalcy may relieve their body image concerns and overcome feelings of inadequacy and unhappiness. Their conscience enables them to be faithful to themselves as authentic beings by self-managing how a plastic world constructs them.

Eagles

For the ancient Greeks, Delphi marked the centre of the world; the point at which two eagles released in opposite directions by Zeus met, collided and fell to the ground. The notion today that patients occupy the centre of health care receives related meaning from recognizing as eagles the patients who elevate self-care to a psychospiritual state of high, energized focus. Eagles achieve this self-transcendence without intoxication. Through immersion in activities like flying – literally rather than metaphorically – they discover personal meaning, direction and purpose in their lives, and help satisfy collective moral interests like harmony. Patient-centred health care has been quiet on the nature and implications for self-care of self-transcendence that is either existential or transpersonal.

Existential self-transcendence is self-care by someone whose sense of self is intact but who becomes conscious of the power of experiencing a larger metaphysical reality. This 'perspective transformation' contributes to self-knowledge and enhances caring for self and others. Nursing theory and gerotranscendence theory have generated studies of such self-transcendence among older adults and ill populations whose suffering has led them to reflect on their lives;

however, ill health is not a requirement for the reflexivity needed for this self-transcendence. Transpersonal self-transcendence takes self-understanding beyond the self by producing a self-forgetful, 'outward loop to inwardness'.[38] One conception of this self-transcendence is the 'ladder to oneness'. It takes people beyond self-boundaries to extended aspects of themselves, the world and the cosmos. An alternative conception – exemplified by Carl Jung's analytical psychology – is the 'spiral to integration'. It casts self-transcendence as a developmental transition that bends back on, and through, itself before ascending to higher levels of experience. However, regardless of whether transcendence is progressive or regressive, dissolution of the distinction in the mind between the self and other produces, as the final step of the developmental ladder, a transpersonal sense of spiritual or emotional union with a single living process. So connected are people to what they are doing, that they experience the world anew and as if there were no separation between themselves and what lies beyond. Transformed from the level of the profane or ordinary to manifestations of the level of the sacred or holy, people feel they have become an integral part of the unified whole or totality of the cosmos.

In psychological terms, this unity has been described as flow – a transpersonal state of consciousness.[39] In this self-forgetful state of deep concentration and complete absorption, people become lost in the intimacy of the moment of peak experience. Ceasing to be conscious of any distinction between themselves and the world, they feel unselfconsciously and fully alive as an integral and vital part of the nature of life. This sense brings them a serene feeling of comfort and belonging. It frees them from the everyday reality of their life and enables them to dwell ecstatically (the Greek word *ekstasis*, meaning 'being outside oneself') in the here and now and experience the immersive joy of being. Recognition of this self-caring state appears heritable[40] and, through neuroimaging, to have a neural basis in the upper rear part of the human brain. Selective damage to this region increases reported self-transcendence,[41] as do some psychopathologies such as dysthymia.[42] However, self-transcendence can and should also be viewed in other than physical dysfunctional terms. The nature of the person, in which the transcendent self is present, makes transcendence possible as a state of being that may signify the highest and most inclusive and holistic state of human consciousness.[36]

Capability and responsibility

Patient-centred health care restricts self-care to protecting the health of patients, as persons whose meaning has been stretched to include the community. In contrast, patients may view self-care as personal behaviour that can extend beyond health. For other people to recognize this behaviour as self-caring however, it is not sufficient for patients to behave any way they want. Self-care is not simply whatever patients choose to make it. Self-care by patients signifies how patients manage their welfare to be faithful to their moral values, interests and capabilities to lead a good life in their particular situation. Therefore, self-care requires authenticity of patients within a life project of cultivating virtues like prudence, temperance and fortitude.[43] In turn, patients' capabilities for this construction of self-care walk the tightrope of constraints on their lifestyle choices. Constraints such as cultural conditioning and biological dependence may moderate moral responsibilities of patients for their health-harming choices. Yet debate continues over the extent to which patients retain self-control and choose how to respond to embodied circumstances, including incentives for personal change.

From the perspective that patients can consciously control their personal actions – even if they cannot control their lived history, social structures and perhaps even brain disease – patients have moral agency. They are not automata and retain capability for self-care. Moreover, despite uncertainty about whether they have a moral right to receive health care from others, they have a right – and responsibility – to self-care. This right-claim is made on *themselves* as persons whose welfare they typically care about – from their perspective. Hence, common among attempts to codify patient responsibilities is a responsibility for patients to self-care for their health. This responsibility fits the need of health systems for patients to help manage rising demand for health care services, control the quality of this care and save costs amid rises in chronic illness and complex comorbidity. The responsibility to self-care may be legally binding as in the German social security code, or be aspirational as in the Scottish National Health Service *Charter of Patient Rights and Responsibilities.*

However, my construction of self-care goes beyond those limited aspirations and those of patient-centred health care, whose communitarian health-centric focus constrains patient agency and de-emphasizes patients' capability to be persons faithfully self-created with stable beliefs and values. Good faith is critical when personal agency and authenticity diverge. Such disjuncture can happen when decisionally competent patients choose to self-care in ways that appear to oppose their prior commitment to practise coherent basic values. Their choice is not truly autonomous if it does not reflect these values and beliefs. However, authenticity is not a sufficient condition for self-care.

Good faith makes behaviour no more self-caring than does patient agency. Acting freely according to one's conscience can produce self-care that is immoral, as when patients harm themselves in ways that reveal less rather than more of their humanity, as a way to cope with personal problems. Beyond acting in good faith, self-caring patients therefore need to develop and exercise additional virtues such as prudence. Off the radar of patient-centred health care, character development enables patients to use their conscience for self-care. I want to position in two groups the capabilities of patients for self-care. The first group relates to self-knowledge. To know their values, which significantly constitute who they are, patients have the capability to get to know themselves. Second, patients can avoid self-pretence, accept themselves and cultivate and realize their further capabilities to construct and implement moral self-care conscientiously in ways they deem appropriate from good character.

Self-knowledge

Self-inquiry and self-knowledge provide insight, as has been long recognized in human history. For example, inscribed on the forecourt of the temple of Apollo at Delphi are two oracular maxims: 'Nothing to excess' and 'Know thyself'. The former injunction speaks to temperance or moderation. 'Know thyself' enjoins people to increase their self-knowledge and know their limitations. Such knowledge may be intrinsically valuable and instrumentally useful. As the physician–philosopher, Moses Maimonides noted, people need to recognize who they are before they can determine who they should become. Emergent self-knowledge further enables people to attend to their limitations rather than fall consistently short, and to be(come) progressively true to what they take their place to be in the everyday world. Only then can they virtuously expect to (re)create, as much as discover, their evolving selves by giving coherent shape to their life. Socrates suggested that the alternative, an unexamined life, is not worth living. Without self-knowledge, he told his student, Alcibiades, people cannot take care of and improve themselves as a precondition to caring for others.

Patient-centred health care's parenthetical interest in patient self-knowledge may reflect the limitations that people face to achieving self-knowledge and using it. People can access some mental states, such as feeling and believing, more easily than others, like knowing. Indeed, most people probably have minimal self-knowledge because, as Thales of Miletus acknowledged, self-knowledge is the most difficult thing in life to achieve. Consistent with the 'self–other knowledge asymmetry model',[44] people want to view themselves positively and block unwanted thoughts and feelings from their consciousness. They lack self-knowledge also when they lack good information about people whose mind is inaccessible to them,[45] and lack appreciation of the moral value of these others.

Even the assumption that the self is knowable has been questioned since at least the time of Heraclitus. According to Eastern philosophies such as Hinduism and Buddhism, the self lacks clear and stable boundaries. From this perspective, people can never really know themselves because they change from moment to moment. In David Hume's empiricist theory of knowledge, they can only experience an ever-changing bundle of sense perceptions that model reality and do not indicate an identity separate from the world. They can be mindful only of their senses in the moment. Mistaking these appearances as knowledge can act against their proper use. In Ovid's *Metamorphoses*, for example, Tiresis had told the nymph Liriope that her son, Narcissus would live to enjoy an old age 'if he shall himself not know'. But he acquired a kind of knowledge of himself as 'no-self'. Narcissus learnt that the reflected appearance with which he was besotted in a still pool was his. He had seen himself or at least his image, which he could not touch and which could not return his love, causing him to waste into a flower. He thought he knew himself but he knew only a simulacrum infected by hubris and the vanity of self-love. Although true self-knowledge is elusive and its appearance is insufficient, this appearance is all that people have. Self-ignorance may produce authenticity as unselfconscious spontaneity[46] but fails to develop people's capability to use virtue to value and care for themselves.

Some cultures, such as the Japanese, tend to value a self-critical focus more than positive self-regard.[47] However, for self-knowledge to produce the destabilizing, progressive effects exemplified in writings by existentialists such as Friedrich Nietzsche, Martin Heidegger and Jean-Paul Sartre, people need both traits including self-acceptance and self-belief that they can self-care in the way they wish. Indeed, they need even the positive version of self-love encapsulated by Aristotle's term, *philautia*, which makes each person their own friend. Facilitated by a positive state of health and awareness, unconditional self-acceptance recognizes the sanctity of life, avoids self-disenchantment and supports people's strength of belief and faith in their right and ability to self-care. It moves them from knowing to doing, while feeling involved and worthwhile in life. This action-guiding, embodied involvement leaves them securely connected with themselves, other people and the environment; bonded to a reality beyond the physical world; and in control of their knowledge and inner experiences. It enables them therefore to recognize that their happiness depends less on external events than on facing their freedom to choose how to interpret and respond to their embodied experience, whatever situated form it may take.

In *Paradise Lost*, poet John Milton expressed this freedom of people, even after a fall into hell, to transcend their physical condition, since: 'The mind is its own place, and in itself can make a heaven of hell, a hell of heaven'. The Austrian Jewish psychiatrist, Victor Frankl and the Russian novelist, Aleksandr Solzhenitsyn made the same point empirically. From surviving internment in Nazi concentration camps, Frankl illustrates how people can choose their attitude in any set of circumstances. To face with nobility the possibilities inherent in their freedom to make this choice can take courage but promises personal growth and meaning. Realizing this freedom and the personal responsibility it generates makes people authentic and constructs a moral path for them to follow. Frankl suggested that people have a will or fundamental drive and capability to find and take this path to meaning, which is larger than they. It gives them a sense of control over their environment and behaviour, so they can address difficult tests as challenges to overcome rather than threats to avoid.[48]

Self-realization with integrity

From self-knowledge and self-acceptance, patients can loosen their social masks, relate authentically to themselves (and others) as persons, and examine and be responsive to their conscience. From a wilful commitment to do what feels morally right, they can question, make, appraise and legitimate the morality of their choices, manage their fear and displace their anxiety.[49] If their conscience then tells them to self-care in a particular way, they will accept this message or risk suffering consequences like guilt. Thus, their conscientious judgements can motivate them to be faithful to themselves and others; for, as Shakespeare's

Polonius counselled his King, Hamlet, 'This above all: to thine own self be true.' Yet, while conscience can govern self-care, virtue is needed to make conscience moral (see Part II).

Patients can cope, say, with having a Body Mass Index outside the normal population range if, in clear conscience informed by their culture and character, they feel comfortable with their body fat and self-manage it freely, in good faith and with prudent compassion. These patients are invoking their conscience – what Horatio in *Hamlet* refers to as the 'mind's eye' – as a private monitor of how honestly self-knowing who they are fulfils their capabilities and interests. Structured by good character, this conscience makes their self-knowledge a moral resource for self-care, entailing personal choices that do not harm others' moral interests and from which, as patients, they have the most to gain or lose.

Conclusion

Patient-centred health care conceives of patient self-care in healthist and communitarian terms. Left ambiguous, moreover, is the meaning of the patient self across increasingly blended private–public spaces. Despite claiming to respect patient autonomy, patient-centred health care also conflates patient agency and authenticity. As a consequence it struggles to recognize as self-care the unhealthy practices that even informed patients of good character can view in good faith as self-caring; and it constructs as self-care the ostensibly healthy practices, such as dieting, that can leave patients feeling bad or worse. There is an unmet need therefore for patients to self-care with integrity on their own terms, guided by clinicians. For example, consider a patient who claims to value their health, yet smokes against the advice of their clinician. This clinician needs to check their understanding of the values and character of the patient; consider how smoking fits this understanding; and, while reflecting on their own values, character and moral interests, close the gap between the patient and themselves to co-create shared benefit. A new care model is needed to accommodate and service this construction of patient self-care.

References

1 Beck U. *Risk Society: Towards a New Modernity*. London: Sage; 1992.
2 Douglas M. *Risk and Blame: Essays in Cultural Theory*. London: Routledge; 1992.
3 Lupton R. *Risk*. Second edition. Oxford: Routledge; 2013.
4 Griffiths C, Foster G, Ramsay J, Eldridge S, Taylor S. How effective are expert patient (lay led) education programmes for chronic disease? *British Medical Journal* 2007; 334: 1254–6.
5 Berzins K, Reilly S, Abell J, Hughes J, Challis D. UK Self-care support initiatives for older patients with long-term conditions: a review. *Chronic Illness* 2009; 5: 56–72.
6 Godfrey C, Harrison M, Lysaght R, Lamb M, Graham I, Oakley P. Care of self – care by other – care of other: the meaning of self-care from research, practice, policy and industry perspectives. *International Journal of Evidence-Based Healthcare* 2011; 9: 3–24.

7 Bycroft J, Tracey J. Self-management support: a win–win solution for the 21st century. *New Zealand Family Physician* 2006; 33: 243–8.

8 Green L, Fryer G, Yawn B, Lanier D, Dovey S. The ecology of medical care revisited. *New England Journal of Medicine* 2001; 344: 2021–5.

9 Porter R. The patient's view. Doing medical history from below. *Theory and Society* 1985; 14: 175–98.

10 Jewson ND. The disappearance of the sick-man from medical cosmology, 1770–1870. *Sociology* 1976; 10: 225–44.

11 Parsons T. *The Social System*. Glencoe, IL: Free Press; 1951.

12 Topol E. *The Patient Will See You Now*. New York: Basic Books.

13 Findley L, Baker M. Treating neurodegenerative diseases. What patients want is not what doctors focus on. *British Medical Journal* 2002; 324: 1466–7.

14 Skrabanek P. *The Death of Humane Medicine and the Rise of Coercive Healthism*. London: Social Affairs Unit; 1994.

15 Le Fanu E, editor. *Preventionitis: The Exaggerated Claims of Health Promotion*. London: Social Affairs Unit; 1994.

16 Collier R. Scared to life. *Canadian Medical Association Journal* 2009; 181: 980.

17 Thomas L. An epidemic of apprehension. *Discover* 1983; 4: 78–80.

18 Barsky AJ. The paradox of health. *New England Journal of Medicine* 1988; 318: 414–18.

19 Schmidt H. The ethics of incentivizing mammography screening. *Journal of the American Medical Association* 2015; 314: 995–6.

20 Heymsfield S, Cefalu W. Does body mass index adequately convey a patient's mortality risk? *Journal of the American Medical Association* 2013; 309: 87–8.

21 Flegal K, Kit B, Orpana H, Graubard B. Association of all-cause mortality with overweight and obesity using standard Body Mass Index categories. *Journal of the American Medical Association* 2013; 309: 71–82.

22 Leventhal H, Brissette I, Leventhal EA. The common-sense model of self regulation of health and illness. In: Cameron LD, Leventhal H, editors. *The Self-Regulation of Health and Illness Behaviour*. Howard: Routledge 2003; pp. 42–65.

23 Reed TJ. Nietzsche's animals: idea, image and influence. In: Pasley M, editor. *Nietzsche: Imagery and Thought. A Collection of Essays*. Berkeley and Los Angeles: University of California Press 1978; pp. 159–219.

24 Kristjánsson K. Phronesis as an ideal in professional medical ethics: some preliminary positionings and problematics. *Theoretical Medicine and Bioethics* 2015; 36: 299–320.

25 Di Castelnuovo A, Costanzo S, Bagnardi V, Donati MB, Iacoviello L, de Gaetano G. Alcohol dosing and total mortality in men and women. *Archives of Internal Medicine* 2006; 166: 2437–45.

26 Ilic D, O'Connor D, Green S, Wilt T. Screening for prostate cancer. *Cochrane Database of Systematic Reviews* 2006, 1; doi: 10.1002/14651858.CD004720.pub3.

27 Gøtzsche P, Jørgensen K. Screening for breast cancer with mammography. *Cochrane Database of Systematic Reviews* 2013, 6; doi: 10.1002/14651858.CD001877.pub5.

28 Kropotkin P. *Mutual Aid: A Factor in Evolution*. London: William Heinemann; 1902.

29 Ovid. *Metamorphoses*. Oxford: Oxford University Press; 1986.

30 Williams B. *Ethics and the Limits of Philosophy*. London: Fontana; 1985.

31 Brehm J, Brehm S. *Psychological Reactance*. New York: Wiley; 1981.

32 Boudon R. Beyond rational choice theory. *Annual Review of Sociology* 2003; 29: 1–21.

33 Vaneigem R. *The Revolution of Everyday Life*. London: Rebel Press; 2001.

34 Ljungdalh AK. Stultitia and type 2 diabetes: the madness of not wanting to care for the self. *Foucault Studies* 2013; 16: 154–74.

35 Russ E, Shedler J, Bradley R, Westen D. Refining the construct of Narcissistic Personality Disorder: diagnostic criteria and subtypes. *American Journal of Psychiatry* 2008; 165: 1473–81.

36 Maslow A. A theory of human motivation. *Psychological Review* 1943; 50: 370–96.

37 Manoloudakis N, Labiris L, Karakitsou N, Kim J, Sheena Y, Niakas D. Characteristics of women who have had cosmetic breast implants that could be associated with increased suicide risk: a systematic review, proposing a suicide prevention model. *Archives of Plastic Surgery* 2015; 42: 131–42.

38 Christoffersen SA. *Transcendence, Self-transcendence, and Aesthetics*. In: Stoker W, Van der Merwe WL, editors. Amsterdam: Rodopi Press 2012; pp. 209–22.

39 Csíkszentmihályi M. *Creativity: Flow and the Psychology of Discovery and Invention*. New York: Harper Collins; 1996.

40 Ando J, Suzuki A, Yamagata S, Kijima N, Maekawa H, Ono Y, Jang K. Genetic and environmental structure of Cloninger's temperament and character dimensions. *Journal of Personality Disorders* 2004; 18: 379–93.

41 Urgesi C, Aglioti S, Skrap M, Fabbro F. The spiritual brain: selective cortical lesions modulate human self-transcendence. *Neuron* 2010; 65: 309–19.

42 Birt MA, Vaida A, Prelipceanu D. Use of the temperament and character inventory personality questionnaire in dysthymic disorder. *Maedica: A Journal of Clinical Medicine* 2006; 1: 29–34.

43 Logan D, Kilmer J, Marlatt GA. The virtuous drinker. Character virtues as correlates and moderators of College student drinking and consequences. *American Journal of College Health* 2010; 58: 317–24.

44 Vazire S. Who knows what about a person? The self-other knowledge asymmetry (SOKA). *Journal of Personality and Social Psychology* 2010; 98: 281–300.

45 Wilson T, Dunn EW. Self-knowledge: its limits, value and potential for improvement. *Annual Reviews of Psychology* 2004; 55: 17.1, 17.26.

46 Feldman S, Hazlett A. Authenticity and self-knowledge. *Dialectica* 2013; 67: 157–8.

47 Heine S, Lehman D, Markus HR, Kitayama S. Is there a universal need for positive self-regard? *Psychological Review* 1999; 106: 766–94.

48 Bandura A. Self-efficacy. In: Ramachandran VS, editor. *Encyclopedia of Human Behavior*. New York: Academic Press 1994; pp. 71–81.

49 Ware O. The duty of self-knowledge. *Philosophy and Phenomenological Research* 2009; 79: 671–98.

4   Clinician self-care

Introduction

It might be argued that clinicians self-care in ways that put patients' welfare first. The Editor-in-chief of the *British Medical Journal* (BMJ), for example, recently cited a contributor to BMJ Careers, who suggested that junior physicians might strike 'for the good of our patients, colleagues, and the NHS'.[1] However, any benefit accruing to patients would be indirect and reflect an underlying need for policy change because the bright light of patient-centred health care casts a vast shadow over clinician welfare.

In illuminating first the welfare of patients, this care puts the welfare of clinicians no higher than second. Through physician acts of last resort, such as strike action, clinicians subordinate their welfare as people – and as moral agents – on whom patients depend. Is it really surprising therefore that, in medicine for example, 'some of the most sensitive and capable physicians today feel like they practice in a medical dark night of the soul'?[2] Unlike owls that love the dark more than the light, they tolerate the dark under the misapprehension that patients benefit from occupying the light alone.

Left wondering what it means to be a physician and, implicitly, a health professional, these physicians languish in role changes to their professional identity. Whether deprofessionalizing them or redistributing their power and resources to other clinicians such as nurses and pharmacists, the changes weaken physicians' autonomy to protect human welfare. Fundamental to these changes has been increased external control over clinical care delivery, which can reduce the ability of physicians and other clinicians to work for patients to the best of their ability without neglecting their own self-care. Economic, medico–legal and patient pressures have been adding to these stresses and need for self-care. Consistent with Chapter 3, I mean self-care in the broad sense of however clinicians choose in moral good faith to serve their own welfare as persons professionally responsible for providing health care.

Feeling depersonalized, some clinicians have chosen to self-care in ways that detract from patient welfare. For example, they have reduced health care to a commodity, exhibiting inappropriate self-interest that takes advantage of patient vulnerability. Such practice includes over-servicing medical care by increasing patient volumes and overprescribing or ordering unnecessary tests to raise clinician incomes. The 2002 Physician Charter[3] sought to reconnect physicians to core values of service. As a code of moral conduct to protect the welfare of patients and populations, however, it has not helped physicians to self-care. It has kept physicians out of the light by obscuring their moral interests.

I am not denying that society takes critical steps to protect clinician welfare, for example by limiting hours of clinical practice out of recognizing the need for clinicians to have time off from work, take vacations, attend conferences and be able to retire. These protections help to expose progress in recognizing the fallacy of the principle of primacy of patient welfare (Chapter 2). Nevertheless, the problem remains that, in medicine for example, aspirational documents such as the Charter reduce physicians to their shadow – a proto-space without physicality – in patient care delivery.[4] The Charter misses the point that physicians' self-care and physician care of patients are not alternatives: these interests are conjunctive and indivisible. If clinicians can care only for others then, as Eric Fromm[5] notes, they cannot care at all, since clinicians who do not care for themselves are ill-equipped to care for patients. In these terms, clinician self-care is important for its own sake as well as for patient care.

In common with the Charter, health reforms in recent decades have been quiet in acknowledging this reciprocity. Emphasizing the welfare of patients and their communities, they say little if anything about the related need to protect the welfare of clinicians. Believing they already serve patients well, clinicians are put under pressure to change the nature and scope of their work in order to shift costs and meet population health goals without necessarily taking the time they need for self-care and patient care. The reforms therefore have tended to marginalize the status of clinicians – and patients – as people; erode independent clinical control over an expanded body of clinical work; prompt clinicians to maximize their bargaining power relative to others, including hospitals and patients; and produce work stresses that commonly manifest in clinician unwellness. This chapter discusses how pressure on clinicians underpins their unwellness and inadequate self-care in the context of their different values, and approaches to attempting to care for themselves. Clinicians, like patients, should be free to self-care in any ethical manner that is faithful to their deep values, within a project of virtue-cultivation and expression – but their siloed duty of care to patients inappropriately constrains this need.

Pressure on clinicians

Restricting clinician autonomy are instruments of managerial authority that shift power from clinicians to managers. To contain costs in the name of 'best practice', a one-size-fits-all approach streamlines the work of group practices, for example through computerized clinical guidelines. Health policy, market-style incentives, and regulations drive clinicians to meet narrowly defined clinical and organizational performance targets; bureaucracy and monitoring hold the clinicians externally accountable for their performance. These changes undermine trust in clinicians' visible ability and commitment to practise humanistic care. At the same time, clinicians are held responsible for patient welfare. Larger social changes also challenge clinicians' capabilities to meet these responsibilities.

The changes include advances in, and expansion of, health information and communication services in quasi-public spaces, and increasing patient literacy. No longer do clinicians monopolize clinical knowledge – and deficits in their knowledge have grown in saliency. Despite the illusion of scientific progress, the last 40 years have generally failed to bring major innovations in clinical care to the bedside. Through the growth of molecular medicine and evidence-based medicine, the new health care technologies have been largely 'fine-tuning and value additions to older ones'.[6] This relative inertia and the unpredictability of clinical care have contributed to erosion of public confidence in, and respect for, clinicians whose work conditions may be poorly understood by many patients. Clinicians strive in this environment to protect their professional authority, relative to respect for patient autonomy. They struggle to meet rising demands and expectations from patients to integrate the myriad pieces of information they present, co-create knowledge and avoid patients' dissatisfaction and complaints.

Work characteristics and demands of clinical roles further test clinicians – and physicians in particular. Facing burgeoning information loads; high cognitive demands, including increasingly complex ethical judgements, for example around end-of-life care options; and reduced 'hands-on' experience with patient care, many physicians – among other health professionals – are working hard for long hours, on average 50 to 60 hours per week when not on call.[7] They may also work irregular hours, including evening or weekend shifts and, under time pressure and other resource constraints, at a quick pace to care for increasing numbers of patients and meet imposed responsibilities for population health care. Pressure to demonstrate regulatory compliance adds to the burden of 'articulation work' that can be hidden but is needed to coordinate and enable activities of growing complexity.[8] Diverting time and effort from patient care, work may be taken home and compete there with obligations for family care and self-care. Women in particular may feel pressure to balance work pressures and family responsibilities and, more than men, be 'constantly beset by divided loyalties and a sense of guilt'.[9]

Other occupational hazards to clinicians can include infections; needle stick injuries; criticism, abuse and other mistreatment from patients – whether deliberate or unintended but experienced by clinicians as oppressive[10] – as well as workplace bullying or harassment. Additional work pressures on clinicians can come from managing emotionally charged and taxing health issues, especially in relation to direct experience of vulnerability and helplessness around patient suffering and death. Physicians in particular may struggle with these issues because not only must they constantly confront existential issues in their work but also 'medicine is the [profession] most likely to attract people with high personal anxieties about dying'.[11] Other personal attributes can also predispose people to choose to become health professionals, find this work stressful and neglect themselves in caring for patients.

Among physicians, these attributes include competitiveness, idealism, perfectionism, compassion, a sense of responsibility, unstable family backgrounds and life adjustment difficulties. These factors contribute to, and exacerbate, low morale, stress and other health risks associated with the high demands that physicians can expect to face at medical school, through residency training and then into professional clinical practice. Emotional dissonance from patients' problems may offer some reprieve but it can also leave physicians feeling guilty. Shame may be felt for any hardening of the heart to pain experienced by patients and, within the unspoken, dark underbelly of health care, even for voyeuristic fascination with it, including an appetite to find illness to heal.[12] Physicians and other health professionals – who are expected to regulate their own emotions; not to care too much or too little; and not inappropriately to expose their own felt vulnerabilities or alarm patients – are at heightened risk of experiencing emotional strain and physical illness. This risk increases without proper social support to brace what one hopes is a deep, 'value-guided commitment for care',[13] yet confidentiality obligations hinder the ability of physicians to share their stress and access this support.

Clinician unwellness and self-care

Clinician dissatisfaction and unwellness are common but often hidden and, as in the H.G. Wells novella, *The Invisible Man*, this imperceptibility can itself stress the clinician. Expected to put patients' welfare first, clinicians seldom talk about these negative states, especially to patients. Clinicians may continue to work when ill, resisting illness, isolation and other work pressures through relatively stable reports of overall career satisfaction in medicine[14] and, for example, audiology.[15]

Paradoxically however, clinicians commonly also derive meaning from clinical work. Most physicians further report being healthy despite unwellness and work stress. In the United States, 'as a group, physicians have healthier lifestyles and lower mortality rates than the general public'.[16] However, suboptimal attention to healthy self-care by physicians who symbolically value health indicates much room for improvement. There is scope, for example, to improve self-reporting by physicians of healthy lifestyle behaviour including preventative care,[17] especially since the physicians practising such behaviour are more likely to recommend it to patients. In turn, role modelling improves patient trust and uptake of health practices.[18] Physician satisfaction has also been associated with improved patient satisfaction,[19] yet chronic stress continues to harm clinicians – especially, physicians and dentists.

Such professionals can find clinical work stressful (as well as rewarding). Beyond the risks of experiencing secondary trauma or empathy fatigue, they commonly feel disgruntled with external demands imposed on them by health systems concerned with managing direct health costs yet acting against timely access to health care. As a twist on a poem by Joseph Malins, *The Ambulance Down in the Valley*, clinicians therefore have become victims who fall off the unfenced cliff.[20] As a long-term outcome of trauma and other work stress, they can eventually suffer burnout as a syndrome characterized by emotional exhaustion, depersonalization and diminished feelings of personal accomplishment. Lacking the visibility and attention it deserves, burnout has become a growing problem from which recovery is difficult.[21] The scale of the problem has been reported for a national sample of physicians in the United States.[22] Almost half of them reported at least one symptom of burnout at work. Despite a low survey response, this prevalence is consistent with reported burnout prevalences ranging from 30–65 per cent across medical specialities[23] and peaking at the front line of medical care.[21,22] Even without burnout, physicians experience increased mental ill-health, such as depression, substance abuse and dependency – especially in relation to prescription drug use for non-medical purposes. These conditions are often stigmatized and can attract disciplinary action from regulatory bodies such as licensing boards, without adequate compassion and support to aid recovery. Other adverse health effects on clinicians include impaired interpersonal relationships, including relationships with family and friends – even suicide[24] – which can spill into work. Female physicians appear especially at risk even though the workplace remains largely oblivious to gender as a predictor of burnout.[21] In turn, unwell physicians risk compromising patient safety and quality of patient care.[24] Yet despite using adaptive strategies, physicians often work when unwell, in part because a culture of professional condemnation and shame has produced a 'conspiracy of silence'.

This silence acts against physicians openly admitting to distress and, if necessary, reporting distress or impairment in colleagues. Failure to speak up resists legal requirements for disclosure, when fitness to practise safely is compromised or uncertain. Those complicit share liability and may wrestle with concern about covering for colleagues whose unwellness is reflected in reduced productivity at work, increased risk of committing serious medical errors and increased absenteeism and early retirement. High job and career turnover characterizes physicians, who are changing jobs within medicine or leaving medicine. When dissatisfied, physicians are less likely to recommend medicine as a career or recommend their own specialty to students, potentially hindering recruitment of the best students.[25]

Shortages of physicians therefore characterize some medical specialities – most notably family medicine, especially in rural and remote areas and the poorest urban areas – and can put unfair pressure on the professions to solve this problem, without adequate resourcing. Health systems also incur significant financial costs in order to train and replace physicians. Overseas trained physicians may provide some respite for host health systems, but these physicians can commonly experience additional stresses compared with local colleagues, including the need to complete unfamiliar, local training and certification requirements. The safety and quality of patient care can be adversely affected. Provider continuity, the relationship with patients, and patient trust can be disrupted; how can physicians 'care for others if we, ourselves, are crippled by ill-health, burnout or resentment?'[26] At the same time, the welfare of clinicians is intrinsically important, not merely instrumentally necessary for them to function well at work (and home) and optimize patient care. Thus, clinicians need to self-care.

As Abraham Lincoln said, 'You have to do your own growing no matter how tall your grandfather was.' Clinicians can self-care alone, however, or under others' supervision. Like everyone else, clinicians should have their own physician and obtain customary health checks. Many physicians lack a regular physician and delay or avoid seeking medical care. Physicians commonly self-diagnose and self-treat despite the risk of compromising their professional objectivity in care delivery, exceeding their limits and not documenting the care they provide or notifying a usual clinician. Cynics might attribute this behaviour to a Zeus complex that seduces some physicians into taking compulsive control of their own health care provision. This psychological complex would delude physicians into believing that their special capabilities justify their exemption from the need for independent care. They may believe they can manage their health problems without 'troubling' a colleague or taking sick leave. Their awareness of limits to medical knowledge and medical care might further motivate them to minimize illness symptoms and delay medical care-seeking. And they might not want to appear weak to themselves and others; feel vulnerable to judgement by a professional colleague; and risk loss of privacy or confidentiality of their medical information, or implications of mandatory disclosure of particular illnesses or impairment for their licensing or credentialing. Such concerns are speculative but, for whatever reasons, physicians in particular may struggle to reverse the roles of clinician and patient; even though as Osler stated, 'A physician who treats himself [*sic*] has a fool for a patient.'

The same warning appears relevant when clinicians treat immediate family members (and even some non-family members such as friends and workmates), except in emergencies or for minor, short-term health problems. However, clinicians' knowledge of their professional peers, and the nature of their work, can widen their choice of and access to health care, with reduced costs. Some health services now enable clinicians to seek help anonymously, which protects their privacy but further cloaks in shadow their health, welfare and care-seeking. How clinicians in this context seek to satisfy their own moral interests is unclear even though, like other people, they need to receive health care from others as well as themselves. In common with the primordial Eros of Greek mythology, clinicians therefore need to emerge from their shadow. They need to join patients in the light and self-care, for example by recognizing the mirror image added to the staff of Asclepius – the emblem of physicians.

How do clinicians 'self-care'?

How clinicians approach self-care varies situationally with their values and identification with competing clusters of health care professionalism.[27] However, the foregoing discussion implies that basic demands from health care professionalism for patient-centred health care have left clinicians insufficiently attentive to, and caring of, their own health needs. For some of these clinicians, this development reveals an identity and practice of non-reflective professionalism. These clinicians seldom 'step back and consider the impact of their behavior on themselves and others'.[28] To the extent that they do look at and after themselves, they self-care in daily cultural routines that adhere to taken-for-granted social norms for self-sacrifice, even if these norms unconsciously oppose classroom-taught values for clinician wellness. These clinicians struggle to self-care until the impact of their work conditions reaches the threshold needed for them to reflect on their practice. In contrast, reflective clinicians vary in their deliberate approach to their work and self-care.

I want to discuss nine values that underpin how – beyond the targeted, structural changes made to support clinicians in the workplace – reflective clinicians may choose to construct self-care and strive to implement it with varying degrees of freedom and success. These values are: conflict avoidance; moral disengagement; 'jealousy'; caring for others; work–life balance; profit maximization; positive attitude; personal and professional development; and authenticity. Non-mutually exclusive, the values vary in their adaptive ability to help clinicians to self-care through optimizing their experience of stresses and pressures of their work. Whether society views the individual values as adequately self-caring for clinicians depends on the extent to which the values can support the development and expression of positive character traits in clinicians and other stakeholders in modern health care.

1 Conflict avoidance

Some clinicians feel deprofessionalized but accept the status quo. They acquiesce to, or accommodate, health policy demands in order to gain social approval, meet financial needs and avoid confronting and risking overt conflict with others. By choosing to comply with bureaucratic rules, these clinicians aim to minimize their own stress and culpability in the event of harm occurring to patients. This passive–defensive approach to self-care tends to eschew concerns that are minor or that cannot be easily resolved in the short term. However, by internalizing their concerns these clinicians can also feel frustrated. They work in the shadow of their secret, hiding how they feel even though this repressive behaviour denies them an authentic identity and social outlet for their dissatisfaction. The same problem characterizes the clinicians who fake compliance to give the illusion of working by society's rules, either to satisfy other people, such as health managers or patients and the public, or to mask the social pressure that they feel to give service to them. This avoidance approach to coping becomes most counterproductive to the full self-care of clinicians when their inner conflict leaves them feeling blocked or trapped at work, and this loss of autonomy eventually burns them out.

2 Moral disengagement

Going beyond clinical distance, other avoidant approaches to coping include related, social cognitive mechanisms of moral disengagement and loss of empathy to prevent vicarious trauma. These mechanisms also free up cognitive resources to facilitate purposeful, complex problem-solving, which can be especially important to clinicians operating under time pressure to deliver efficient, objective and effective health care to patients. Clinicians also avoid moral self-sanctions by maintaining intact their self-image as ethical persons.[29] Yet, moral disengagement and lack of empathy are ultimately maladaptive. They isolate clinicians and predict their unethical behaviour by permitting clinicians to distance themselves from, or rationalize, past harm and act unethically toward patients who need clinicians to understand and empathize with their illness experience and accompany them through it.

3 'Jealousy'

Chapter 2 discussed the Munch picture, *Jealousy*, where the front male figure, which I interpreted to symbolize a clinician, appears unhappy. The largeness of his face suggests that he also craves attention. Does it defy credibility for *Jealousy* to depict a clinician who, as per the title of the picture, is 'jealous'? On my reading, the clinician may indeed be jealous – though not of patients. Rather, the clinician may be jealous of the progress that others collectively have made vis-à-vis clinicians' own deprofessionalization, loss of professional autonomy and frequent unwellness. You might respond that an ideal clinician is other-focused and that the emotion of jealousy indicates a pathological egoism inconsistent with health care professionalism. However, jealousy is merely the dark side of the empathy commonly ascribed to clinicians and, besides, justified jealousy is not necessarily a vice.

Akin to righteous indignation, justified jealousy can be a rational and morally appropriate response to dispossession – a social force necessary for a productive life of personal and professional integrity and welfare. Such a life is a balanced life, wherein 'all the different emotions add their diverse tones, at the right times and in the right proportions, to life's symphony'.[30] Following Aristotle's golden mean, jealousy that can be morally justified is a virtue, balanced between the narratives of too much and too little sensitivity to undeserved treatment. From this perspective, stable and self-respecting clinicians cannot be expected to be without jealousy when warranted. Jealousy then is their duty. They *should* be jealous of developments such as bureaucratic managerialism and increased control by a modern laity distrustful of their service orientation and clinical leadership of health care. These changes amplify the sacrifices made by clinicians, without producing an 'apparent compensatory increase in satisfactions',[31] and threaten clinicians' sense of justice and moral agency, their need to care and flourish, and the public interest. Moreover, these clinicians are in the best of company since the justifiably jealous clinician is an apotheosis. As John Donne[32] preached in his sermon at the marriage of Margaret Washington almost 500 years ago, 'Jealousie that implies care, and honour, and counsell, and tendernesse, is rooted in God, for God is a jealous God and his servants are jealous servants.' Maimonides questioned whether God, being God, has attributes, but if clinicians, like God, sometimes act in ways that can be construed as jealous, they are rightly jealous at losing something important.

4 Caring for others

Openly resisting unwellness-producing changes to health care professionalism are the clinicians who are nostalgic for a 'professionalism of old' grounded in traditional values such as increased clinician autonomy and beneficence. Regarding clinical practice as personally rewarding, these clinicians embrace it as a selfless vocation and, to that end, sacrifice their self-interests. Their compassion for patients is satisfying and reduces clinician turnover.[33] Yet, there is a risk of self-denying clinicians reducing their self-care to an indirect effect of feeling good about helping others – an important feeling for sure, but one that unhelpfully anaesthetizes clinicians' insensibility to their own independent need for health and welfare. Doing nothing directly to meet their moral interest in receiving care can be maladaptive for clinicians. Most at risk are those working often alone and in relative professional isolation, for example as solo clinicians or in small practices – especially in rural and remote areas.[27]

Many clinicians in academic life and, more generally the 'ruling class' of individuals, groups and organizations whose status in medicine is elite, yearn to resurrect clinician agency for personal care. Another clinician group comprises activist clinicians. Acting often in organized forms, they commonly accept conditions such as the heavy workloads needed to fight politically for, and achieve a social contract model of, professionalism that serves the health and well-being of all members of society. At the same time these clinicians demonstrate problem-focused coping by committing to fundamental, system-level change in health care as a social good, which can ameliorate the social conditions that impact negatively on justice and equity in areas such as indigenous health, mental health, tobacco control and climate change. The clinicians who identify with this model commonly receive specialized training in public health, health policy or social and community health. Beyond the commitment of all clinicians to address social determinants of health, they may volunteer their time, for example in free clinics; work as advocates and educators to improve systemically the health and living conditions of the sickest patients and most disadvantaged population groups; resist external regulatory oversight; and actively attempt to improve clinicians' conditions and standards of work. From all of this effort these health care professionals reap intrinsically motivating rewards such as pride and gratitude.

5 Work–life balance

Sir William Osler recommended that, 'The young doctor should look about early for an avocation, a pastime, that will take him away from patients, pills, and potions ...'.[34] And certainly, amid growing concern in society about declining 'quality time' for self, family and community, there are lifestyle clinicians. They freely choose, on the basis of their core values, to balance their clinical workload against pursuing other activities, commitments and interests, which they find meaningful as an aid to growth and re-creation in their personal and family lives. These interests may include actively participating in enjoyable, goal-directed leisure activities but also other, provident forms of work – both unpaid, such as raising children or looking after sick relatives, or paid, as exemplified by academic medicine. The last option can offer flexible opportunities for clinicians to combine their clinical practice with formal teaching, service and research in scholarly areas of personal and public interest. This mix of activities may allow the progressive option of spending some work time at home and blending personal self-care into work time, for example by taking regular breaks and remaining socially connected during the day with other people at work and with valued ones outside the office.

When important to clinicians, such balance may be sought in some periods of life but not others, so as not to inhibit ambitions such as career development. Constructing work and home life as not necessarily competing spaces, clinicians may take time out from work to participate in forms of non-work or play, such as hobbies or other creative leisure activities outside the workplace. Accommodation of these personal interests may require these clinicians to accept flexible work options in disciplines like family medicine. These options may include part-time work, occupying specific practice niches to minimize patient demand, and job sharing. Taking these options, as Bertrand Russell explained, can produce self-care by enabling clinicians to live fully; relieve their work strain, including the status anxiety of 'affluenza'; be compassionate, but not overwhelmed, by caring within boundaries;[33] and re-energize themselves. Yet these outcomes do not come without costs. Work–life balance may require shifting work tasks onto others, and depend on clinicians exploring experience of new resources while maximizing experience of current resources such as a partner who helps to balance work and family commitments. Properly organized however, work–life balance may achieve a healthy, fulfilling and productive life; advance patient care; and satisfy organizational discourses over control of work.[35] James Wallman[36] describes this common lifestyle as 'experientialism', a value-based and identity-enhancing system that emphasizes doing rather than the 'stuffocation' of having.

However, Oxford scholar, Theodore Zeldin[37] goes further. Suggesting that work–life balance, in itself, does not prevent work from being oppressive, he encourages people to strive to develop new ways of work that do not feel to them like work. Making work personally satisfying – by softening a rigid division between work and non-work – is instrumental therefore to an ideal work–life balance. From this perspective, clinicians can *choose* to practise health care and, rather than merely cope with its demands, actively celebrate the privilege of managing them with others in the here and now in a positive way. This celebration, explains Ronald Epstein,[38] requires 'engagement, being fully present in one's work, and deriving meaning and nourishment from it even in moments of conflict, unhappiness, tough decisions and difficult tasks'. What allows that engagement, he suggests, is resilience. Pause for thought also comes from Alain de Botton's observation that work–life balance is largely a myth because work worth doing tends to unbalance life; and people each have only one life in which

to use this impulse as a resource to grow and find personal meaning and fulfilment in work.

6 Positive attitude

There is scope for clinicians to self-care, in part, by managing their work
through gratification for it. These clinicians optimally experience even objectively adverse work conditions. They achieve this autotelic state of 'flow' by
understanding that what ultimately counts is their conscious attitude toward
these conditions. Thus, they develop a positive attitude by finding meaning in
their work and its purpose of supporting health and healing. With pride and
humility, they recognize as a gift their opportunity to work as clinicians. They
understand that this opportunity is a privilege, a prize that makes them privy to
some of the most intimate aspects and moments of patients' lives. For the gains
that patients, in turn, have made, these clinicians are not jealous but happy; just
as John Keats explained his pain in *Ode to a Nightingale* by stating, '"Tis not
through envy of thy happy lot,/But being too happy in thine happiness.' This
positive mindset is conducive to work engagement and intrinsic satisfaction as
well as material rewards, elevated social status and power. Especially with role
convergence and democratization of health care, the privileges can become nor-
malized and invisible to clinicians. However, personal and professional development (see below) can enable clinicians to acquire self-knowledge; rediscover
who they are, not merely what they have; and celebrate their identity. Regardless of whether they can ameliorate their work conditions, gratitude then helps
to produce self-care through maintaining a positive attitude that balances rather
than erases work stress.

Counterbalancing empathy fatigue, this positive attitude among clinicians
includes compassion satisfaction and the inner spiritual freedom and ability to
'smile at the raging storm'.[39] As discussed further in Chapter 7, clinicians generally choose to smile – but not to trivialize the terror of the storm, derive pleasure
from the pain it can inflict or detest this pain. Rather, they smile courageously
to acknowledge the pain without holding it. They reframe the pain to give resil-
ient meaning and purpose to their work and quality of life, improve their mood,
and even reduce their own risk of physical morbidity and mortality.[40] Other
ways in which clinicians may demonstrate a positive attitude include humour
such as joking and laughter. However, particularly in hospitals and the most
stressful clinical work spaces, including the emergency room, the operating
room and critical or intensive care units, there is also backstage humour that is
black – and its moral appropriateness can be ambiguous.

Also known as gallows humour, black humour between the clinicians who
share the same demanding work environment makes performative lightness of
patients' tragic situations. Examples include describing dying patients as
'heading to the ECU' (external care unit) or the 'departure lounge' for 'celestial
transfer'. The absurdity of the incongruity of this black humour[41] can make
callous fun of defenceless patients 'approaching room temperature', and expose

a dark underbelly of health care. Paradoxically, however, such humour may put virtue into action. Katie Watson[42] suggests how. She distinguishes the 'jolly bully' from the overwhelmed clinician struggling to survive an oppressive workplace. For the latter clinician, use of black humour is not necessarily unethical when, without harming patients or their families, it is sparingly used as a distraction or a device to defuse despair. The humour is virtuous when, without wounding the patient, it helps clinicians regulate their emotions, not feel enslaved and mitigate their vulnerability and defencelessness. Relief theorists, most notably Herbert Spencer[43] and Sigmund Freud,[44] have suggested how humour can produce these benefits.

They propose that humour can be cathartic by releasing intolerable tension or pressure. Humour can also heal by facilitating social connectedness with peers. Both mechanisms can enable clinicians to stay sane in the sometimes-insane work environment of health care practice, and indeed feel spurred to virtuous action. In these terms, clinician humour and its object – human suffering – can have positive meaning. Yet, the medical workplace, laments Watson, is less funny than it once was. Other coping mechanisms have become preferred methods of self-care by clinicians, who perhaps should not be permitted to work in highly stressful environments for long periods. While black humour tightropes rough seas, she suggests that 'perhaps the hand wringing has gone too far' and too readily dismisses the need of clinicians, as people, for empathy in order to self-care in a brutal environment.

Facilitating and reinforced by a positive attitude, strategies such as humour are not inconsistent with Stoic behaviour that manifests qualities such as dignity. Indeed, Cicero[45] suggested that virtue is sufficient for a happy life since the virtue of doing the morally right thing produces a positive outlook and prevents work stress from deflating happiness. Epictetus had similarly advised in his second century manual of ethical advice, the *Enchiridion*, that 'Men are disturbed not by things, but by the principles and notions which they form concerning things.'[46] And Victor Frankl demonstrated that – no matter how dire the circumstances – people retain the power to decide how to respond.[47] Thus, while some clinicians take their work beyond unhealthy limits, others construct their work as an enjoyable and rewarding way to express personal aspirations (like moral integrity, through an ethic of work as a civic responsibility) and realize a sense of achievement and purpose. Even if clinicians depend on their work to furnish these benefits, and this work is stressful for them at times, it can confirm a positive self-image that suffuses non-work parts of their lives and is an organizational asset.

7 *Personal and professional development*

At times, despite their vocation, clinicians – as persons – may self-care by privileging aspects of their life other than health. Even when they value health highly, their reasons may vary. Arguably, health is less intrinsically good than morally neutral since it can produce benefit or harm. In these terms, clinicians may value health as a personal adaptive state, existing in the absence and presence of identifiable disease, creating space for them to do good. Other clinicians value health for its own sake. Either way however, clinician health can be a core professional value to which many clinicians commit through healthy living. Every day they may aim to make healthy choices such as to get adequate sleep, eat nutritious food as part of a balanced diet, maintain a healthy weight and exercise regularly.

Such clinician self-care has generally not been included in medical training or emphasized in professional practice, which inculcates self-sacrifice. Moreover, models for health maintenance to prevent clinician burnout have been poorly documented, although the situation is improving. Professional groups such as the Royal College of Physicians and Surgeons of Canada now expect physicians to 'demonstrate a commitment to physician health and sustainable practice'[48] and physicians can learn about how to recognize and manage work-related stress. Clinicians are increasingly encouraged to commit to lifelong learning for personal and professional development.

This undertaking can require clinicians to acquire and apply virtues and skills in their work and life. One reason that virtue can facilitate self-care is that clinicians protect their psychological resources when they are true to themselves and can trust themselves to do the right thing because it feels right to them – rather than from the self-restraint that characterizes the clinician of continent character, who acts well despite the desire to act otherwise.[49] Relevant skills for clinician self-care include time management and strategies for reflection, such as reflective writing; meditation; and other techniques for self-awareness and integrative stress management, like mindfulness of present moment experience. The clinicians who most value their own health are especially likely to have usual clinicians, as noted above, and obtain timely access to independent health care to protect or improve their health.

Participation in professional support networks can, in turn, facilitate clinicians' professional development. Clinicians can work collaboratively in teams, and voluntarily receive supervision or 'educative mentoring'. Clinicians may also receive debriefing for professional support and clinical development, and participate in peer support groups – such as Balint groups or Schwartz rounds – to acknowledge and examine their own emotions and manage with equanimity the paradox of caring and health professionalism. Other development options include taking educational opportunities for lifelong learning from attendance at professional meetings and training courses; participating in health advisory and referral services and educational activities including projects for quality improvement and research; and acquiring life skills, such as mindfulness meditation. Beyond these forms of self-regulation, clinicians may participate in external regulation programmes such as accreditation.

Lastly, let me elaborate on how teamwork can facilitate self-care. In much health care practice, physicians work relatively independently as discrete professionals. However, cooperative and collaborative working by physicians and other professionals in teams can facilitate clinician self-care, for example in the patient-centred medical home. Expressing civility and cooperation in the workplace, teamwork and communication can directly strengthen clinician self-care by providing a vehicle for clinicians to interact productively with their peers in complex and challenging work environments. Their energized interaction can furnish information and collegial support, for example by anticipating care needs and sharing workload. Indirectly, teamwork can enhance clinician self-care by coordinating and optimizing patient care that is safe and effective. In turn, clinicians can self-care through interactions with patients. Some 14–17 per cent of physicians have been found to self-disclose selected personal information to patients during routine office visits, which can meet physician needs for self-care while potentially strengthening physician–patient relationships.[50,51] However, disclosure risks disrupting patient care despite good intentions, for example by silencing patients' stories.

8 Profit-maximization

Clinician self-care depends on clinicians receiving from private and public payers what they perceive to be fair remuneration for their services. However, entrepreneurial health professionals, who own clinical practices or work within small partnerships, have a business mindset that emphasizes the importance of this remuneration. Encouraged to compete financially with each other, they accept high workloads, increased financial responsibility, and high stress levels (at work and across the work–home divide) to minimize utilizing health care resources and maximize their work income (or profit).

At the start of this chapter, I cast clinician profit-maximization as a dark space that tends to entice clinicians to act against business ethics and their own self-care. A Midas-like drive to accumulate material wealth can become dehumanizing and isolating, lead clinicians to feel spiritually empty, and feel unjust to the public, without whose support they would not be able to work as clinicians. Moreover, the profit imperative can get in the way of clinicians caring properly for themselves and their patients. Yet, entrepreneurial professionalism in health care can also create pockets of light within a dark space; like stars in the night sky. For example, receiving a high income cannot directly increase subjective well-being but it can help clinicians to achieve instrumental goals that are moral or at least morally neutral. These goals can be financial, such as to pay off a large student debt, and professional, such as to unlock productivity and meet socially sanctioned, patient-defined needs. Such rewards may in turn ameliorate negative events such as work stress and help clinicians to feel successful.

To boost their income in work environments that they consider competitively healthy, these clinicians may opt to work long hours. They may also develop new technologies; take on non-clinical leadership roles like a clinical directorship; or, within clinical medicine, enter a procedural specialty such as orthopaedics. The last choice is especially attractive when private work is available and clinicians can achieve high, billable work volumes for services yielding high profit margins. Income opportunities are lower for physicians in non-procedural specialties, such as paediatrics and primary care. However, even in primary care, physicians can earn high incomes when retainers enable them to deliver luxury or concierge care to elite subscription patients who are able and willing to pay for it. Also financially attractive to clinicians can be adjunct incentives. These include target payments like special payments, recruitment incentives, bonus payments for achieving performance targets specified by pay-for-performance programmes, and profit-sharing after minimizing costly medical interventions.

9 *Authenticity*

Whichever socially endorsed approach the clinician takes, their self-care requires them to reflect on the ethics of their professional behaviour and motives. Mindful that their role persona is merely part of who they are and can complicate attempts to know themselves, they need to strive for self-knowledge and accept themselves. They further need to be faithful to their values around their preferred model of health care professionalism and to themselves as people. Clinician self-care is not merely therefore about the abilities of clinicians; more than a form of expertise, it requires them to realize and actualize the person they already are. This requirement needs clinicians to self-author challenging but achievable personal goals, align their style of working with these values and empower themselves by acting consistently on these values. For example, consider the clinician who self-exposes vulnerability and cries in communicating bad news to a patient. The emotional openness of this behaviour is not necessarily unprofessional. Self-caring for the clinician, the tears may be appreciated by the patient; just as Oliver Twist received 'such kind and gentle words, and such tears of sympathy and compassion, that they sank deeper into Oliver's soul, than all the sufferings he had ever undergone'. The alternative is to act inauthentically. Yet, Søren Kierkegaard explained that when people seek to become someone they are uncomfortable with, either they will fail – and spurn themselves – or succeed, but at the cost of abandoning their true selves. Either way, they will despair.

Conclusion

Environmental, work-related and personal factors interact to put clinicians under high pressure. To put the welfare of patients first, these clinicians have contributed to creating for themselves a shadowed space that masks their own and others' ability to recognize this predicament and its consequences for them and their patients, and manage both. Most importantly, their unwellness in the space of patient-centred health care lacks visibility, is prone to inattention and tends to compromise patients' interests. Clinicians are taught to accept their conditions of working for patients on the grounds that, compared with patients, they have a lesser claim on receiving care – from themselves, no less than others. However, this belief compartmentalizes patient care as a service industry without accounting for how it interacts with clinician welfare. Even when clinicians recognize and seek to treat their own unwellness and problems associated with their work, they are disadvantaged relative to projects caring for patients. The inegalitarian stage on which clinicians and patients play scripted roles disrespects the personhood and relational interdependence of both parties; misses the point that the role of clinician does not remove neediness; and puts clinicians and patients at risk of deterioration and harm from reduced safety and effectiveness. Also hidden can be how clinicians reflect or not and act on their need to self-care on the basis of their values, understanding of health professionalism, and duty of care to patients. This chapter has discussed values that underpin how clinicians seek to self-care. Morally praiseworthy values – such as caring for others, humour, work–life balance, a positive attitude, personal and professional development, and authenticity – inform my model of person-centred health care in Part II.

Notes

1 Godlee F. More sinning than sinned against. *British Medical Journal* 2015; 351: h6369.
2 Pellegrino E. Character formation and the making of good physicians. In: Kenny N, Shelton Q, editors. *Lost Virtue: Professional Character Development in Medical Education.* (*Advances in Bioethics, Volume 10*). Oxford: JAI Press 2006; pp. 1–15.
3 ABIM Foundation, ACP-ASIM Foundation, European Federation of Internal Medicine. Medical professionalism in the new millennium: a physician charter. *Annals of Internal Medicine* 2002; 136: 243–6.
4 Gothill M, Armstrong D. Dr. No-body: the construction of the doctor as an embodied subject in British general practice 1955–97. *Sociology of Health and Illness* 1999; 21: 1–12.
5 Fromm E. *The Art of Loving.* New York: Harper and Row; 1956.
6 Mittra I. Why is modern medicine stuck in a rut? *Perspectives in Biology and Medicine* 2009; 52: 500–17.
7 Williams ES, Rondeau KV, Xiao Q, Francescutti LH. Heavy physician workloads: impact on physician attitudes and outcomes. *Health Services Management Research* 2007; 20: 261–9.
8 Sawyer S, Tapia A. Always articulating: theorizing on mobile and wireless technologies. *The Information Society* 2006; 22: 311–23.
9 Symonds A. Emotional conflicts of the career woman: women in medicine. *American Journal of Psychoanalysis* 1983; 43: 21–37.
10 Smythe E. The violence of the everyday in healthcare. In: Diekelmann NL, editor. *First, Do No Harm. Power, Oppression and Violence in Healthcare.* Madison: University of Wisconsin Press 2002; pp. 164–203.
11 Nuland SB. *How we Die.* New York: Knopf; 1994.
12 Sontag S. *Regarding the Pain of Others.* London: Penguin; 2003.
13 Larson E, Yao X. Clinical empathy as emotional labor in the patient–physician relationship. *Journal of the American Medical Association* 2005; 293: 1100–6.
14 Landon BE, Reschovsky J, Blumenthal D. Changes in career satisfaction among primary care and specialist physicians, 1997–2001. *Journal of the American Medical Association* 2003; 289: 442–9.
15 Severn M, Searchfield G, Huggard P. Occupational stress amongst audiologists: Compassion satisfaction, compassion fatigue, and burnout. *International Journal of Audiology* 2012; 51: 3–9.

16 Frank E. Physician health and patient care. *Journal of the American Medical Association* 2004; 291: 637.

17 Kay M, Mitchell GK, Del Mar CB. Doctors do not adequately look after their own physical health. *Medical Journal of Australia* 2004; 181: 368–70.

18 Frank E, Dresner Y, Shani M, Vinker S. The association between physicians' and patients' preventive health practices. *Canadian Medical Association Journal* 2013; 185: 649–53.

19 Haas JS, Cook EF, Puopolo AL, Burstin HR, Cleary PD, Brennan T. Is the professional satisfaction of general internists associated with patient satisfaction? *Journal of General Internal Medicine* 2000; 15: 122–8.

20 Malins J. A fence or an ambulance. 1895; Available at: www.poemhunter.com/poem/the-ambulance-down-in-the-valley. Accessed 7 July 2014.

21 Linzer M, Levine R, Meltzer D, Poplau S, Warde C, West C. 10 bold steps to prevent burnout in general internal medicine. *Journal of General Internal Medicine* 2013; 29: 18–20.

22 Shanafelt T, Boone S, Tan L, Dyrbye L, Sotile W, Satele D, West C, Sloan J, Oreskovich M. Burnout and satisfaction with work–life balance among US physicians relative to the general US population. *Archives of Internal Medicine* 2012; 172: 1377–85.

23 Soler JK, Yaman H, Esteva M, Dobbs F, Asenova RS, Katic M, Ozvacic Z, Desgranges JP, Moreau A, Lionis C, Kotányi P, Carelli F, Nowak PR, de Aguiar Sá Azeredo Z, Marklund E, Churchill D, Ungan M. European General Practice Research Network Burnout Study Group. Burnout in European family doctors. *Family Practice* 2008; 25: 245–65.

24 Wallace J, Lemaire J, Ghali W. Physician wellness: a missing quality indicator. *Lancet* 2009; 374: 1714–21.

25 Wetterneck TB, Linzer M, McMurray JE, Douglas J, Schwartz MD, Bigby J, Gerrity, MS, Pathman DE, Karlson D, Rhodes E. SGIM Career Satisfaction Study Group. Worklife and satisfaction of general internists. *Archives of Internal Medicine* 2002; 162: 649–56.

26 Irvine C. The ethics of self-care. In: Cole T, Goodrich T, Gritz E, editors. *Faculty Health in Academic Medicine*. Totowa, NJ: Humana Press 2009; pp. 127–46.

27 Castellani B, Hafferty FW. The complexities of medical professionalism. In: Wear D, Aultman J, editors. *Professionalism in Medicine. Critical Perspectives*. New York: Springer 2008; pp. 3–23.

28 Coulehan J. You say self-interest, I say altruism. In: Wear D, Aultman JM, editors. *Professionalism in Medicine. Critical Perspectives*. New York: Springer 2006; pp. 103–27.

29 Bandura A. Moral disengagement and the perpetration of inhumanities. *Personality and Social Psychology Reviews* 1999; 3: 193–209.

30 Kristjánsson L. Why persons need jealousy. *The Personalist Forum* 1996; 12: 163–81.

31 Reed R, Evans D. The deprofessionalization of medicine. Causes, effects and responses. *Journal of the American Medical Association* 1987; 258: 3279–82.

32 Potter GR, Simpson EM, editors. *John Donne, The Sermons of John Donne. Vol. 3*. Berkeley: University of California; 1962.

33 Post S. Compassionate care enhancement: benefits and outcomes. *International Journal of Person Centered Medicine* 2011; 1: 808–13.

34 Osler W. The medical library in postgraduate work. *British Medical Journal* 1909; 2: 925–8.

35 Muhr SL, Pedersen M, Alvesson M. Workload, aspiration, and fun: problems of balancing self-exploitation and self-exploration in work life. *Research in the Sociology of Organizations* 2013; 37: 193–220.

36 Wallman J. *Stuffocation*. London: Crux; 2013.

37 Zeldin T. How work can be made less boring. *British Medical Journal* 1999; 310: 163–5.

38 Epstein RM. Realizing Engel's biopsychosocial vision: resilience, compassion, and quality of care. *International Journal of Psychiatry in Medicine* 2014; 47: 275–87.

39 Schoch R. *The Secrets of Happiness*. London: Profile Books; 2007.

40 Huppert FA, Whittington JE. Evidence for the independence of positive and negative well-being: implications for quality of life assessment. *British Journal of Health Psychology* 2003; 8: 107–22.

41 Kant I. *Critique of Judgment*. New York: Hafner; 1951.

42 Watson K. Gallows humour in medicine. *Hastings Center Report* 2011; 41: 37–45.

43 Spencer H. The physiology of laughter. *Macmillan's Magazine* 1860; 1: 395–402.

44 Freud S. *Jokes and their Relation to the Unconscious*. New York: W.W. Norton; 1905.

45 Steel CEW, editor. *The Cambridge Companion to Cicero*. Cambridge: Cambridge University Press; 2013.

46 Epictetus, editor. *The Enchiridion*. Raleigh, NC: Generic NL Freebook Publisher; 1996.

47 Frankl V. *Man's Search for Meaning: An Introduction to Logotherapy*. Boston: Beacon Press; 1963.

48 Royal College of Physicians and Surgeons of Canada. The CanMEDS 2005 Framework. 2005; Available at: www.royalcollege.ca/portal/page/portal/rc/common/documents/canmeds/framework/the_7_canmeds_roles_e.pdf. Accessed 17 October 2014.

49 Baumeister RF, Exline JJ. Virtue, personality, and social relations: self-control as the moral muscle. *Journal of Personality* 1999; 67: 1165–94.

50 Beach MC, Roter D, Rubin H, Frankel R, Levinson W, Ford D. Is physician self-disclosure related to patient evaluation of office visits? *Journal of General Internal Medicine* 2004; 19: 905–10.

51 McDaniel SH, Beckman HB, Morse DS, Silberman J, Seaburn DB, Epstein RM. Physician self-disclosure in primary care visits: enough about you, what about me? *Archives of Internal Medicine* 2007; 167: 1321–6.

5 Patient care of the clinician

Introduction

Everyone needs care – not only patients. In general, all people depend on approval from others to feel less isolated, less vulnerable and more cared about within social relationships, than they otherwise would. In common with patients, clinicians therefore need to receive care too. However, can and should patients help to provide it and besides, who is the clinician? The clinician can be compared to the cat-woman in the photograph *Io Gatto* (Cat and I). Merging a self-portrait of the Italian photographer, Wanda Wulz, with a portrait of one of her family cats, Mucincina, the image conflates their dual identities – yet viewers can immediately recognize the cat-woman as a fiction masking her personal identity. Likewise, the *persona* of the clinician is a role representation, a performative identity which obscures the clinician as a *person* despite, in so doing, actually drawing attention to the ambiguity of the person of the clinician. Thus, the cat-woman symbolizes depersonalization of the clinician whose real nature is concealed but who seems caring and – in common with the patient – needs to secure care directly, as well as through care-giving, for the benefit of both parties.

Clinicians and health systems have been slow to recognize and respond to this need – inclusive of caring – of clinicians within health care. Even slower to develop has been general recognition of the need and capability of *patients* to help provide it. Chapter 4 discussed the need for self-care of clinicians as 'second victims' who may access support through systems, including peers and primary affiliates, outside health care. As key members of health care teams, however, patients may signify an additional resource for providing this support. Sceptics might challenge this suggestion as impractical. They may argue that I ask too much of patients in a world where – as W.H. Auden's poem, *Musée des Beaux Arts* depicts, in Pieter Breughel's *Landscape with the Fall of Icarus* – 'everything turns away' from human suffering. Not even all clinicians are caring toward patients, without this detachment always bothering patients, so why should society expect patients, who may be sick and typically pay for health care, to be caring toward clinicians? Besides, not all patients are modern patients.

However, suggested Joan Tronto,[1] caring is a 'species activity' fundamental to the human condition and behaviour, including how patients relate to others.

Consistent with this perspective of care as a normative concept, patients frequently need to demonstrate their moral development. In a world that still has an appetite for uncaring behaviour, they have within them the potential to distinguish themselves as caring by caring for others, including clinicians. The least socially advantaged patients tend most to display this moral preference.

Yet all patients who are capable of caring can be motivated to care about their clinician, in part because of the personal nature of health care. From necessity, health care draws patients into close contact with their clinician in a therapeutic alliance. Especially in negotiated moments of embodied intimacy – when patients feel exposed and vulnerable – they can struggle not to care about, and for, their clinician and thereby not to self-care. Patients can derive satisfaction, and even therapeutic benefit, from doses of care-giving to clinicians whilst having the most to gain or lose from the quality and safety of the care they help their clinician to offer them. Patients, like clinicians, may also suffer from repressing naturally occurring empathy toward clinicians. Yet patients tend to be exempted from care-giving to clinicians or have it received with ambivalence. Patients become 'good' in the eyes of others by meeting role expectations to behave themselves and make the most of their clinical care. Care of clinicians is not expected from patients even if they can, and want to, offer it to clinicians who need it.

From my perspective however, there is an unmet need and opportunity to delineate the scope and significance of the care that can and sometimes does take place from patients to clinicians, frequently for potential, shared benefit. When clinicians reject or lack interest in patient care-giving, they devalue themselves and patients as people and moral agents who may want to care for clinicians whose performance affects them. Certainly, patients are vulnerable. However, failure to respect their capabilities and preferences to care for clinicians undermines respect for their autonomy – including policies encouraging patients to claim their voice in health care – and exposes an underlying presumption of inequality that is patronizing and disrespectful. Devaluing patients as caregivers nevertheless typifies clinician-centric language in modern health care. Terms such as 'provider continuity', 'medical error' and 'pay-for-performance' fail to recognize patients as moral agents and primary health care workers who co-produce, not merely consume, health care for themselves and others.

Four phases of care potentially characterize patients, no less than others,[1] and give them more credit than they typically receive.[2] These phases overlap and distinguish *care* as a practice that builds on but tends to overshadow *caring* as a felt and valued state of attentiveness. Caring, the first phase of care, entails 'caring about' the clinician, whom the patient recognizes as needing care,[3] and wants to give it, for example out of gratitude. The patient can care about the clinician through attentiveness to, and recognition of, the clinician's interest in receiving care from others. Phases two to four relate to care practices that build on, or occur without, the emotional investment of phase one. Phase two is 'care-taking from' the clinician, by which the patient who accepts clinical care honours the clinician who, in turn, has reason to feel an intrinsic sense of satisfaction. The third phase is 'taking care of' the clinician as a human being in whose welfare the patient has a personal interest. The patient accepts a need and obligation to care. This phase blurs into the fourth phase, 'care-giving', which entails adequately resourced patients acting on this felt responsibility by providing care directly to the clinician. This care-giving involves patients, no less than clinicians, as partners-in-care who, to the extent of their capabilities, exhibit felt kindness as 'a way of knowing people beyond our understanding them'.[4] When enabled to know clinicians as people, patients are further empowered to offer and give care to clinicians.

This chapter advocates for patient care-giving as an underdeveloped resource. Reasserting the ideal of the patient–clinician relationship as a mutual, reciprocal engagement maintained by feedback loops, I want to discuss the potential value of patient care-giving to clinicians and patients. Since patients tend to lack recognition and be underutilized as caregivers to clinicians in patient-centred health care, I will also consider barriers and capabilities to patient care-giving. I will suggest that exercising this capability to care is liberating for the patient within the limiting power of the clinician–patient relationship, although with this freedom comes moral responsibility. Clinicians in this context need to partner with patients to address these issues.

Value of patient care-giving

While prudence is needed in responding to patient care-giving, clinicians repudiating this care can harm themselves and patients. Through self-abnegation, clinicians forego the kindness that, as human beings and vulnerable clinicians, they need. They harm themselves when they turn patient kindness into a forbidden pleasure. This sacrifice may help clinicians to feel safely detached but it can also leave them rueful, alienated and lonely since, consciously or otherwise, clinicians and patients share a need to feel valued. As William James explained, 'The deepest craving of human nature is the need to be appreciated.' At the same time, 'no one can know his own beauty or perceive a sense of his own worth until it has been reflected back to him'.[5]

This construction of the patient as a mirror, reflecting care from the clinician, contributes to how clinicians see themselves. In their relations with other people, clinicians need and deserve recognition and gratitude. The independence of autonomous clinicians is a liberal fiction. Relations of mutual interdependence require them to receive care in order to provide it on the battleground of occupational hazards like burnout, unwellness and exposure to dying and death. Paradoxically, therefore, clinicians' power in health care makes them vulnerable. Rather than diminish their position, and further weaken or infantilize them, patient care-giving can benefit them (and patients) sociophysiologically by reducing allostatic load from stress and low morale.[6] Clinicians can protect or regain their strength through patients, as care-partners, self-caring and creating over time a relational space for joint care and healing. Indeed in small rural and remote areas, dual relationships with patients may be unavoidable since patients may easily become colleagues or friends. This space answers the need of clinicians to live a normal life. Patients enable clinicians to feel alive and important by caring for them in their own way.

Clinicians can and do learn much from their patients (and informal caregivers) as well as by being patients. From patients' stories about their experiences with health care, clinicians learn not only about how well the health system works but also about their patients and themselves. As William Osler observed, 'the best teaching is that taught by the patient'. As a form of care, it can take place in clinical practice; educational and training programmes including curriculum design and development and classroom teaching, including assessment; research activities; and quality improvement. For example, people with Parkinson's disease (PD) have served as expert contributors to European PD consensus standards of care[7] and European PD Guidelines for Physiotherapeutic Care.[8] Through such forms of involvement, patients can teach and support clinicians-in-training and clinicians by sharing lived experience, while developing their own knowledge and skills. These patient contributions and outcomes erode a tradition where 'the patient, though treated with courtesy, has usually been little more than a medium through which the clinical teacher taught'.[9] Patients can now model caring as a respectful component of multi-dimensional thinking about matters of importance.[10]

Through their own 'caring thinking', clinicians become aware of, and responsive to, their emotions and those of patients and deliver improved care. Through accepting care-giving from patients, clinicians strengthen their connectedness to these patients and the therapeutic potential of a more equal, clinician–patient relationship in which patients – no less than clinicians – can benefit from care-giving to a clinician more powerful than they.

Patients can benefit because the power of the clinician can arouse patients' respect and reverence. Responding to the human weakness of the strong clinician humbles patients and kindles patients' empathy and care-giving. Illuminating the clinician, this care-giving can be care-receiving for patients. It frees patients to fulfil their own humanity, delight in this fulfilment; love themselves, as an antidote to the observation, by Jacques Lacan, that people tend to hate themselves; and grow their trust in clinicians, increasing patents' moral authority and concordance. Thus, care-giving by patients does not oppress or sacrifice their own welfare for the good of clinicians. Rather it liberates and strengthens patients, less to repay any debt than to realize their ethical project to lead a good life.[11] This generosity, or at least benevolence, rewards patients emotionally and respects their freedom to respond to a common need for care. It helps patients to avoid an excessive focus on themselves, normalize their illness and find meaning and purpose outside their own satisfaction; that is, live joyfully for something beyond themselves. Not allowing patients to give care to clinicians acts against these outcomes by limiting patients' ability to see and respect clinicians as people behind, or beyond, their professional role.

Many patients need to show such respect to others to feel fully connected and human through maintaining healthy and productive social relationships.

Caring for others, including clinicians, enables patients to lead a life of fairness and reciprocity within their community. As emphasized by the Stoics, the self is a communal self. In the absence of individuals caring for others on the basis of rationality and affection, there can be no sense of community. Neighbourliness functions as 'cultural cement' that pastes them into society.[4] Beyond this communalism, patients can feel shame or even guilt when denied their biologically programmed need to reciprocate care. They may feel embarrassed by their loss of autonomy. In caring for the clinician in their own way, patients can alleviate this feeling; actualize their inherent sociality as persons who need to engage with others to feel fully human; and, as Jean-Jacques Rousseau suggested, recover their natural disposition for kindness. Thus, through care-giving, patients look for survival and their very being. If care-giving cannot achieve this existential ideal, it can at least furnish satisfaction from a sense of mutual benevolence within a broad commitment to reciprocity. This commitment reflects social norms that sociology and evolutionary and social psychology construct through theories of social exchange and rational choice. Patients may further benefit instrumentally from enabling clinicians to be well, feel appreciated and provide the best health care they can.

Barriers to patient care-giving

Two key sets of barriers act against clinicians and patients achieving this positive value from patient care-giving. The first relates to the vagueness and self-reliance of clinicians as persons to care about. As noted at the start of this chapter, clinicians tend to present themselves to patients as obscure subjects. At least outside small communities, including rural and remote settlements, patients 'see' and know their clinicians poorly as people. These clinicians choose to remain indistinct within the shadows of patients, and their own professional role. The personhood of individual clinicians, while not completely hidden to patients, has become generalized into a role or persona of strength and independence that resists care from dependent patients. I acknowledge that, symptomatic of an improving balance between rationality and emotions, such detachment has weakened. In New Zealand, a cross-sectional survey of young physicians found that over one-third of those with Facebook accounts had not activated their privacy options, making personal information publicly available.[12] Yet, in clinical care, even when the same clinician cares longitudinally for patients, patients typically catch but a glimpse of the clinician as a person open to receiving care from them. Society cautions clinicians not to remove their professional mask and expose their vulnerability by sharing personal experiences or showing much emotion. Caution is exercised ostensibly to avoid upsetting patients, altering professional boundaries or discrediting the profession. However, privacy is counterproductive when excluding patients acts against them trusting their clinician as they silently wonder, 'Who is the clinician who asks me to open myself to their care?'

To partner with clinicians as moral equals – with whom they have a professional but intimate relationship – patients need to know them. In common with the sculptor, Pygmalion, patients need moral life breathed into what they care for, and only by knowing and trusting the character of the clinician can this enlivenment take place. To get to know clinicians, especially when the relationship with the clinician develops over time, patients need them to weave relevant life experiences into their patient care and present this tapestry with emotional openness and gentle honesty, within limits that prevent over-sharing and benefit both parties. Only then can patients and clinicians know each other as people – their general traits but also the values and beliefs informing their decision-making – without harming anyone. As Erich Fromm[13] explained, 'To respect a person is not possible without *knowing* him [*sic*]; care and responsibility would be blind if they were not guided by knowledge. Knowledge would be empty if it were not motivated by concern.' The veil of darkness over the clinician adds to and can frustrate concern among patients wanting but unable to know and choose the clinician on whose welfare they depend. Frequently, patients can only render the clinician distinct by filling in shadow.

The legendary potter, Butades of Sicyon, modelled a relief from the outline that his daughter had traced of the shadow, on the wall, of her sleeping partner. So too do patients give form to the shadow of the clinician. From how the clinician appears, they imagine what the clinician is like in different respects. They infer elements of the content of the clinician's mind from how the clinician behaves. However, just as Chema Madoz's photograph, *Tenedor cuchara*, reveals a spoon with a fork shadow, such inferences can misrepresent objective reality. Though patients may create a positive fiction, which enables them in a situation of uncertainty to care about the clinician, this fiction is less desirable than openly communicating reason and emotion. When clinicians share life experiences relevant to the patient's presenting problem, then just as the touch of Rapunzel's tears reopened the eyes of the blinded prince in the Grimm brothers' fairy tale, so too can the clinician revealed as a person enhance the patient's ability to give and receive care from this person.

The second set of barriers to patient care-giving relate to the role of the patient. Since patients may be sick or worried they are sick, have less power than clinicians, and directly or indirectly are likely to be paying for their health care, should society expect them to be caring toward clinicians? Indeed, might *uncaring* patient behaviour even assist clinicians when it is clinically revealing, for example of patient stress, lack of coping ability or mental illness? A patient's uncaring behaviour in this situation may remind clinicians that the patient has greater health needs than they; offer insights into the nature, cause and significance of these needs; and provide cues as to how best to manage them. Through the virtue of grace, clinicians can further recognize uncaring behaviour as part of what it means to be human and, in that context, be enabled to accept their own imperfections.

Perhaps most important, however, is concern that expecting patients to be caring toward clinicians increases patients' vulnerability – not least to exploitation by clinicians and to physical and mental harm. Patient care-giving may also reduce patients' limited autonomy to reject treatments offered by the clinician, and increase risks of inappropriate intimacy and crossing legal and ethical boundaries designed to protect patients and clinicians. Nevertheless, health concerns do not burden all patients and even those who suffer from these concerns may choose to express their felt need and capability to care about their clinician. In this context, clinicians, practising by consent of patients, may be mainly concerned for themselves. They may fear patients sharing the power they have traditionally controlled, and exercising 'powers of the weak'.[14] Illustrating how even innocuous acts of patient caring can discomfort clinicians is clinician uncertainty over how to respond to patient 'thank you' messages and, in particular, gift-giving. All caring from patients can be described as 'care-in-gift'[15] but patient gift-giving typically refers to the patient transferring a present or some other item of value.

Such gift-giving is common; although, in Canada, for example, neither the code of ethics of the medical profession nor this profession's charter for physicians advises physicians on how to respond. In contrast, the American Academy of Pediatrics states that 'accepting modest gifts [from patients] does not involve a serious conflict'. It acknowledges that such gifts from patients are mostly benign, being typically intended to express gratitude. Patients likely gain satisfaction from their gift-giving – even though pleasure is not their prime motivation for offering the gift – and refusal of the gift could offend them.[16] Patients will repress their gratitude which, in the words of William Arthur Ward, must feel 'like wrapping a present and not giving it'. In rural communities, moreover, which can be characterized by close interactions across social settings, gift-giving may take place within friendships that develop before the roles of patient and attendant clinician. There is also a risk of double standards; how can clinicians choose not to accept a modest gift from a patient, yet accept corporate 'gifts', such as those from pharmaceutical companies and other health-related commercial organizations?

Of concern to clinicians, nevertheless, is that a patient with low self-esteem may give a gift out of desire for friendship or to curry special treatment. Since ancient times – and especially since the writings of the philosopher, Thomas Hobbes, and his critics, such as David Hume and Adam Smith – the authenticity of kindness vis-à-vis self-interest has been contentious. And gift-giving can foster patient transference – that is, predispose patients unconsciously to transfer a need for a desired or past relationship – and, in turn, clinician countertransference. To avoid self-harm and harming the patient, clinicians carefully manage these emotions that, in themselves, are normal and can be important components of therapeutic relationships. Clinicians are likely therefore not to accept a substantial gift, especially if offered to create or maintain a 'medicine of friends', in which the physician attends to a patient who is also a friend, or who sees the physician as a friend. Accepting such a gift risks changing a boundary crossing into a boundary violation, and may compromise clinical judgement and the ability to provide effective clinical care; for the same reasons, clinicians are typically advised not to treat family or friends for other than minor ailments. Additional reasons that clinicians may be reluctant to accept gifts and other care from their patients include not recognizing their own care needs as clinicians, not wanting to remind themselves of their human vulnerabilities (or failings) and those of their patients, and not valuing care from patients highly. Once associated largely with male clinicians, these motivations to resist patient care-giving are now also recognized to characterize female clinicians.[4] And clinicians may reject patient care to maintain their privileged social status, authority and control over patients. As a way forward, the American Medical Association's Report of the Council on Ethical and Judicial Affairs recommended that physicians adhere to the 'rule of transparency'[17] by only accepting gifts they would feel comfortable disclosing to colleagues or the public in the best interest of the patient–physician relationship.

Nevertheless, 'the shift from potentially harmless dual relationships or activities outside the professional service to sexual relationships is a slippery slope'.[18] Acceptance of patient care mandates caution when it risks leading to sexual contact. Especially for psychiatrists but also clinicians such as family physicians (who likely treat more psychiatric patients than do many psychiatrists[19]) sexual involvement with patients introduces legal issues, including the risk of criminal prosecution, as well as ethical dilemmas. The latter include uncertainty around whether a patient can freely give informed consent to sexual involvement with their clinician. Whether or not a clinician can morally have sexual contact with a former patient is ambiguous. Agreement is lacking on the acceptable time interval between ending a clinician–patient relationship and beginning sexual contact.

Should patients therefore give up on care-giving to clinicians? I believe that it is a sad indictment on Western society that, in general, clinicians have become wary of patient care-giving – and suspicious, even phobic in this modern age stained by competitive individualism, that patients' acts of seeming kindness belie egoistic motives. Such fearful suspicion constructs patients – as Thomas Hobbes suggested in the *Leviathan* – into covetous beasts who care for nothing but themselves. At the same time, clinicians, like all people, need to receive kindness and are no different from other human beings in commonly feeling deprived of it. They want the kindness of care but may resist it; and they may also be uncomfortable with the patients who are unkind toward them. Withstanding the need for clinicians to self-care and be properly cared for by their health system, patients are part of this system and, as people, can and arguably should care for clinicians to the extent they are able.

Capabilities

'Piglet', said A.A. Milne, 'noticed that even though he had a Very Small Heart, it could hold a rather large amount of Gratitude.' So too, patients are mostly capable of caring in some way. There are patients, quintessentially with psycho-pathologies or sociopathologies, who exhibit profound deficits of empathy and impairment of emotional and motivating moral judgement. However, besides being rare in the general population, such people may still be capable of giving care to others even if they do not care about them. Moreover, they may even be capable of empathy, as exemplified by some Nazi leaders expressing concern for, and agitation over, the welfare of their pets (an irony that makes these men all the more culpable for their barbarous actions). Compared with these human monsters, most patients are much less constrained of course in their capability for caring and can and do demonstrate appropriate emotional responding despite ill-health.

Indeed, research shows that even at the end of life, sick patients may have and express feelings like gratitude and concern for others.[20] For example, in qualitative interviews, 13 hospice patients in two New Zealand cities described their experience of such personal concern and caring, including empathy and closeness to others, including their clinician.[21] These patients chronicled how they benefitted from acting on their capability to give care. They helped to co-produce health care – as when they used humour to help the clinician to communicate with them in difficult circumstances – which added meaning to their own life. Gratitude for their care, even in life's darkest hours, could promote compassion, act against feeling depressed and foster courage.

Such caring can take place because adversity can furnish wisdom – as Samuel Taylor Coleridge's poem, *Quae nocent, docent* (What hurts, teaches) explains. This insight is particularly important because, added Albert Camus, 'What we can or cannot do, what we consider possible or impossible, is rarely a function of our true capability. It is more likely a function of our beliefs about who we are.' Clinicians have confirmed this observation by describing care-giving from dying patients without loss of social authority. Abraham Verghese,[22] for example, has recounted patients at the end of life engaging him in clinical rituals of symbolic significance – as much for his benefit as theirs – because of who these patients are and how they sustain their self-worth. Hence, even very sick patients can and want to care for clinicians who can be motivated to gain from it when patients benefit from giving modestly of themselves. And most patients are not yet at the end of their life.

Most patients are community members who, from the premise that power is embedded in people, share common human resources to care situationally for their clinicians. The physician, William Pickering[6] noted, 'the invaluable natural reservoir of kindness in a community'. And increasing patient literacy and narrowing social distances have grown the capability of many modern patients to care for clinicians with whom they share deep values, blend social roles and become increasingly alike over time.[23] These social forces have also actualized sociobiological responses to receiving care. The mirror neuron system and other neurobiological mechanisms appear to prime patients to share physiology with, and reciprocate care to, those who exhibit care to them. From this perspective, patients share care and this sharing itself is caring. Their self-care and care from others, such as clinicians, empower them to return care to those with whom they share the centre of health care.[24]

Patients can care for clinicians by caring for themselves, partnering with them during visits and supporting research and community initiatives to improve system and service delivery design. In many countries, the Choosing Wisely initiative, for example, is engaging and educating patients to work with clinicians in their communities to identify and recommend clinically appropriate health care in individual situations. Patients also formally provide care to peers in associations and support groups that may meet face-to-face or online to provide information, advice and support. Informally, patients care indirectly for clinicians through providing dependent family members and friends with instrumental, emotional and informational care beyond the norm of social expectations. Often this care is ongoing, becomes routine and is invisible. Strengths-based approaches that support resilience and resourcefulness mitigate the often-significant personal costs to informal carers, whose character disposes them nevertheless to care with clinicians as joint partners. Often having their own health problems that make them dependent, the carers may be cared for at the same time. Indeed, their need for and receipt of care qualify them particularly well to reciprocate care. Feminist scholars have long pointed out how those most lacking power disproportionately perform the work of caring that society requires of them.

Patients are able to care for clinicians by being good patients, or at least not bad patients. It seems reasonable to expect that, in the absence of the causative influence of disease, patients will not generally opt to be 'bad' patients.[25,26] In an age when reports of aggression and violence by patients have been increasing,[27] patients will not be uncaring toward clinicians. Uncaring patients – who have also been variously described as problem patients or as difficult, hateful, heartsink, dysphoric or challenging patients – display negative, rule-breaking behaviour. Encounters with these patients, although clinically meaningful, can 'kindle aversion, fear, despair or even downright malice in their doctors'[28], and this response can demoralize these patients and harm their health care. Four types of dysfunctional patients present frequently in modern general clinical practice: the so-called 'dependent clinger', 'entitled demander', 'manipulative help rejecter' and 'self-destructive denier'.[29] Beyond such patients are those who exhibit widespread, subtle forms of dehumanization such as bad manners – the ubiquitous 'violence of the everyday'. Modern society routinely condones such behaviour despite its risk of negative consequences, such as recipients' feeling of reduced moral worth. Might patients be enabled to become aware of, and reflect on, this behaviour, and minimize it contextually through new patterns of socialization?

Meanwhile, most patients can also display positive forms of simple caring for their clinician. Through self-care, patients may reduce inappropriate demand for services from clinicians, clinics and the health system. In patient–clinician interactions, most patients can genuinely and respectfully: greet clinicians; enquire as to their well-being; listen with open-minded interest; use body language to show that they care about what the clinician says and does; express gratitude; and show loyalty, for example by returning to see the same clinician. By comparison, it may be more demanding, yet still feasible, for most patients to: give relevant information to the clinician; show concern and compassion for the clinician as a person whose vulnerability may manifest in tiredness or unwellness; contribute to constructive dialogue and creative, deliberative decision-making; and forgive the clinician for real or perceived minor errors. Even for the clinician whose equivocal and minor improprieties appear uncaring, the patient may be able to care by using the so-called 'as if' approach. Giving the benefit of the doubt to the clinician, and thereby self-caring and protecting the relationship, the patient imagines and acts as if the clinician is caring.[30] Evident here is the patient's autonomy – the ability to make independent and purposeful choices about their behaviour in health care, including care-giving to the clinician.

Patient obligations

Is care-giving morally elective however, rather than morally required or able to be prescribed – at best a virtuous act rather than a moral obligation? If so, then patients might opt not to care for their clinician, perhaps because of unwellness or the clinician has been uncaring toward them or not conspicuously caring. One reason for the salience of the last concern is that, at least in large cities, patients increasingly interact with clinicians as moral strangers; patients encounter from a distance, 'not a known and trusted face, but teams of professionals who are neither names nor faces'.[31] Nevertheless, from the perspective that caring is a collective (public) responsibility, I believe that patients still have a moral responsibility to be caring toward clinicians to the extent that patients have this moral capability and may already demonstrate it, for example in their self-care. Moreover, patients may be the best people to care for clinicians at times when clinicians most need care. Consider, for example, an online photo of an Emergency room physician in tears, minutes after losing his young patient.[32] A colleague might help this physician compose himself before he attends other patients, but those patients would then undermine this support if they complain about mundane issues such as waiting an unnecessarily long time.

I acknowledge that for patients to care for others can take energy that these patients may need to conserve when very unwell. Caring is not necessarily a finite resource but limitations of health, time and other resources prevent patients from giving everyone equal care. In general therefore, capable patients choose how to care rather than whether to care. For them to be caring is their natural impulse; their personhood calls on them to exercise it in everyday life. Even at the end of life, they may discover personal strength. Signs of social withdrawal may be balanced by a final surge of energy – empowering the empathic bond of a light touch or a compassionate look. As Edvard Munch wrote, 'I felt as if invisible threads led from your eyes into my eyes and tied our hearts together.'[33] Expenditure of this energy may be constructed less as emotional labour than as a salutary form of flow, and for most patients death is not near, increasing their obligation to care and self-care.

From care-giving to clinicians, patients too may benefit, as noted above. However, regardless of any instrumental gain, patients derive an obligation for care-giving from their character, emotion and rationality as self-legislating persons,[34] since 'autonomy without responsibility is not autonomy'.[35] Virtues such as justice may also call them to this responsibility. Consistent with reciprocity theory,[36] they cannot pass to others an obligation 'to give back the good that is given to them'[37] without denying their own personhood. Put simply, patients are morally obligated to accept and act, within the scope of their capabilities, on the mutual need to provide care to others, including clinicians, and accept from them their caring and concern. This perspective argues against Talcott Parsons' functionalist notion that the 'sick role' of 'sanctioned deviance' exempts patients from obligations to perform usual 'well roles' beyond cooperating with the clinician to improve their health. Yet, cooperation itself implies caring, unless patients' weakness empowers them to become exempt. At the same time I ask less of patients than Edmund Pellegrino and David Thomasma imply, in stating that, 'The patient, like the physician, has all the obligations of any human being in a moral relationship with others.'[38]

For such reasons, patients in reality are not completely exempted by society from being caring toward others. Some patient charters, such as Scotland's National Health Service *Charter of Patient Rights and Responsibilities*, have specified patient responsibilities, but these responsibilities have in the main been 'specified weakly in terms of how patients should *not* act'.[39] For example, patients should not act in a violent or aggressive manner toward others. The few positive acts expected explicitly of patients include attendance for appointments on time or giving timely notice to the clinic if they know they will be late; sharing honestly all potentially relevant information with the clinic; paying bills on time (in the absence of a special arrangement); and treating clinic staff (and other patients) with due dignity and respect. The last expectation relates to respect for the personhood and expertise of clinicians, for example by having realistic expectations of them.

Patients are generally obligated therefore to avoid choosing to behave indelicately, and to try to take positive actions toward clinicians. Despite the paucity of explicit guidance from the health professions on the scope and importance of patient responsibilities for care-giving to clinicians, patients are socialized to act in ways that affirm moral and social values that belong to them or at least their communities. Consistent with Erving Goffman's theory of ceremony, and the model of patient-centred health care, the minimum action typically required of patients is situated adherence to the ritual order of tacit rules of clinician–patient interactions. Adherence to these rules – including conventional greetings and other 'minor courtesies, civilities and signs of deference' – satisfies basic social requirements for the interactions[40] to function cooperatively as a social and micro-political performance.[41] Halley Faust[42] exemplifies this perspective by defining kindness as a way of helping others without necessarily feeling empathy or compassion. Such kindness may be construed as behaviour as simple as good manners that, whether genuine or strategic, are 'ethically equalizing'.[43] Martin Seligman and colleagues[44] add that lack of sincerity is unimportant because imagining and acting 'as if' sincerity were momentarily present create a social space within which people can interact respectfully. However, while believing that patient care-giving can help to stabilize the ethics of moral encounters[45] beyond charters and codes of conduct, I am inclined to resist attempts to make allowances for inauthentic behaviour.

From my perspective, constraining patients' care-giving obligations to the ceremonial order of social etiquette is much too limiting. Most people want others to commit to their well-being and be genuine in their expressions of care, and they can generally recognize sincerity when they encounter it; for example, people can commonly distinguish an authentic Duchenne smile from the appearance of a manufactured fake. In turn, clinicians – no less than patients – may view surface-level acting as mechanical, disingenuous and undermining of the ability to demonstrate benevolence in good faith. Inauthentic patient care-giving may also even damage the health of patients; for example, among men with coronary disease, so-called non-enjoyment smiles have been reported to be positively associated with transient myocardial ischaemia.[46] And insincerity is often unnecessary to the extent that people can make the effort to change the emotions they experience. For example, I view Hans Vaihinger's 'as if' approach as a form of deep acting that can modify emotional experience and produce sincerity.[30] Jennifer Scott[47] therefore further suggests that, 'Although authentic compassion could be described as heartfelt in nature, it is also our professional duty as health care providers.' My view is that no one can be obligated to feel caring emotions like gratitude that some people, in some situations, feel more easily than others. However, I do not think that expecting patients to be as caring as they can be asks too much of them. Patients, for example, ought to try to feel grateful when they express gratitude, or at least refrain from impoliteness. All I am asking is that patients, like other people, be faithful to their own values and beliefs even though these beliefs may be mistaken, and cultivate and exercise virtues like politeness and honesty.

I acknowledge that, in practice, ill-health and power asymmetries in clinician–patient relationships can act *against* patient candour, and *for* a 'sense of place' in relation to others for the sake of rapport-building and conflict avoidance.[48] However, honesty and truthfulness are not tactlessness and recklessness; and for that reason, people may be caring by remaining silent, and indeed often must do so.[49] Role convergence and reduced social distances also characterize clinician–modern patient relationships. Therefore, whatever people say, they should mean. Dissimulation is the last resort, despite Amiens' assertion, in Shakespeare's *As you Like it*, that 'most friendship is feigning'. As idealist as my position may appear, it is softer than that espoused by philosophers such as Immanuel Kant, for whom veracity is an unconditional duty derived from reason.

Conclusion

Clinicians rob patients of their personhood when they deny patients' felt or expressed need and capability to recognize and care about them as persons. Patients should be enabled to show authentic care to clinicians as a form of sincere benevolence, which makes possible a mutual experience of joining and a unifying sensation of wholeness. For the same reasons, it is not enough for patients to care about clinicians but not communicate this care to the extent they can. Thus, the vulnerability of patients cannot necessarily exclude them from this qualified, moral obligation. There will always be some patients who cannot care in any way about anyone or anything, owing to physical or mental incapacity or both. However, when patients can care in some way, and most already demonstrate this capability in relation to themselves and others, there is no good reason to excuse them – as persons – from a moral obligation to be caring toward their clinicians. Clinicians cannot enforce an obligation for patient care-giving but they can facilitate its fulfilment. They can model caring behaviour and positively reinforce care-giving from patients who have been encouraged to act on the basis of their conscience. Such changes nevertheless indicate a need to move beyond the model of patient-centred health care.

Notes

1 Tronto J. *Moral Boundaries: A Political Argument for an Ethic of Care.* New York: Routledge; 1993.
2 Segal J, Baum NH. Lessons to be learned from patients and colleagues. *Medical Practice Management* 2014; July–August: 49–52.
3 Frankfurt H. The importance of what we care about. *Synthese* 1982; 52: 257–72.
4 Phillips A, Taylor B. *On Kindness.* London: Penguin Books; 2010.
5 Powell JJ. *The Secret of Staying in Love.* Niles, IL: Argus Communications; 1974.
6 Pickering W. Kindness, prescribed and natural, in medicine. *Journal of Medical Ethics* 1997; 23: 116–18.
7 *European Parkinson's Disease Association. The European Parkinson's Disease Standards of Care Consensus Statement,* 2011 (Updated 2012); www.epda.eu.com/en/publications/parkinsons-consensus-statement/.
8 Keus M, Munneke M, Graziano M, Paltamaa J, Pelosin E, Domingos J, Bruhlmann S, Ramaswamy B, Prins J, Struiksma C, Rochester L, Nieuwboer A, Bloem B. On behalf of the Guideline development group. *European Physiotherapy Guideline for Parkinson's disease.* 2013; www.parkinsonnet.info/media/11928217/eu_20physiotherapy_20guideline_20pd_review_2020131003-1.pdf.
9 Spencer J, Godolphin W, Karpenko N, Towle A. *Can Patients Be Teachers? Involving Patients and Service Users in Healthcare Professionals' Education.* Newcastle: The Health Foundation; 2011.
10 Lipman M. *Thinking in Education.* Cambridge: Cambridge University Press; 2003.
11 Gunderman RB. *We Make a Life by What We Give.* Bloomington, IN: Indiana University Press; 2008.
12 MacDonald J, Sohn S, Ellis P. Privacy, professionalism and Facebook: a dilemma for young doctors. *Medical Education* 2010; 44: 805–13.
13 Fromm E. *The Art of Loving.* New York: Harper and Row; 1956.
14 Janeway E. On the power of the weak. *Signs: Journal of Women in Culture and Society* 1975; 1: 103–9.
15 MacBride-Stewart S. Motivations for the 'gift of care' in the context of the modernization of medicine. *Social Theory and Health* 2014; 12: 84–104.

16 American Academy of Pediatrics, Committee on Bioethics. Policy statement: pediatrician–family–patient relationships. Managing the boundaries. *Pediatrics* 2009; 124: 1685–8.

17 American Medical Association (AMA). Report of the Council on Ethical and Judicial Affairs. CEJA Report 4-A-03. Gifts from patients to physicians, 2003.

18 Alexander C, Charles G. Caring, mutuality and reciprocity in social worker–client relationships: rethinking principles of practice. *Journal of Social Work* 2009; 9: 5–22.

19 Campbell DC, Searight HR. Physician–patient sexual contact: ethical and legal issues and clinical guidelines. *Journal of Family Practice* 1993; 36: 647–53.

20 McPherson C, Wilson K, Murray MA. Feeling like a burden: exploring the perspectives of patients at the end of life. *Social Science and Medicine* 2007; 64: 417–27.

21 Janssen A, MacLeod R. Who cares for whom? Reciprocity of care at the end of life. *Journal of Palliative Care and Medicine* 2012; 2: 129.

22 Verghese, A. A doctor's touch. TEDGlobal; 2011; www.ted.com/talks/abraham_verghese_a_doctor_s_touch

23 Buetow S, Jutel A, Hoare K. Shrinking social space in the doctor–modern patient relationship: a review of forces for, and implications of, role convergence. *Patient Education and Counseling* 2009; 74: 97–103.

24 Kunz G. *The Paradox of Power and Weakness: Levinas and an Alternative Paradigm for Psychology.* New York: State University of New York Press; 1998.

25 Stokes T, Dixon-Woods M, Williams S. Breaking the ceremonial order: patients' and doctors' accounts of removal from a general practitioner's list. *Sociology of Health and Illness* 2006; 28: 611–36.

26 Kelly MP, May D. Good and bad patients: a review of the literature and a theoretical critique. *Journal of Advanced Nursing* 1982; 7: 147–56.

27 Naish J, Carter YH, Gray RW, Stevens T, Tissier JM, Gantley MM. Brief encounters of aggression and violence in primary care: a team approach to coping strategies. *Family Practice* 2002; 19: 504–10.

28 Groves JE. Taking care of the hateful patient. *New England Journal of Medicine* 1978; 298: 883–7.

29 Strous RD, Ulman AM, Kotler M. The hateful patient revisited. Relevance for 21st century medicine. *European Journal of Internal Medicine* 2006; 17: 387–93.

30 Buetow S. Caring about the clinician who appears uncaring: the 'as if' approach. *Journal of Evaluation in Clinical Practice* 2015; 20: 957–60.

31 O'Neill O. *Autonomy and Trust in Bioethics.* Cambridge: Cambridge University Press; 2005.

32 Wible P. Heart-wrenching photo of doctor crying goes viral. Available at: www.idealmedicalcare.org/blog/heart-wrenching-photo-of-doctor-crying-goes-viral-hereswhy/. Accessed 2 December 2015.

33 Torjusen B. *Words and Images of Edvard Munch.* London: Thames and Hudson; 1989.

34 Stern R. *Understanding Moral Obligation: Kant, Hegel, Kierkegaard.* Cambridge: Cambridge University Press; 2012.

35 Draper H, Sorell T. Patients' responsibilities in medical ethics. *Bioethics* 2002; 16: 335–52.

36 Roberts CA, Arugute MS. Task and socioemotional behaviors of physicians: a test of reciprocity and social interaction theories in analogue physician–patient encounters. *Social Science and Medicine* 2000; 50: 309–16.

37 Marcinowicz L, Pawlikowska T, Konstantynowicz J, Chlabicz S. New insight into the role of patients during medical appointments: a synthesis of three qualitative studies. *Patient* 2014; 7: 313–18.

38 Pellegrino ED, Thomasma DC. *For the Patient's Good: The Restoration of Beneficence in Health Care*. New York: Oxford University Press; 1988.

39 Schmidt H. Patients' charters and health responsibilities. *British Medical Journal* 2007; 335: 1187–9.

40 Baldwin J. A social requirement theory of moral obligation [dissertation]. Indiana: Notre Dame; 2008.

41 Fisher S. Doctor–patient communication: a social and micro-political performance. *Sociology of Health and Illness* 1984; 6: 1–29.

42 Faust H. Kindness, not compassion, in healthcare. *Cambridge Quarterly of Healthcare Ethics* 2009; 18: 287–99.

43 Warren M. What should and should not be said: deliberating sensitive issues. *Journal of Social Philosophy* 1996; 37: 163–81.

44 Seligman A, Weller R, Puett M, Simon B. *Ritual and its Consequences. An Essay on the Limits of Sincerity*. New York: Oxford University Press; 2008.

45 Strong PM. Minor courtesies and macro structures. In: Drew P, Wooton A, editors. *Erving Goffman: Exploring the Interaction Order*. Cambridge: Polity Press 1988; pp. 37–56.

46 Rosenberg EL, Ekman P, Jiang W, Babyak M, Coleman RE, Hanson M, O'Connor C, Waugh R, Blumenthal JA. Linkages between facial expressions of anger and transient myocardial ischaemia in men with coronary artery disease. *Emotion* 2001; 1: 107–15.

47 Scott J. Authentic compassion. *Obstetrics and Gynecology* 2013; 122: 148–50.

48 Intachakra S. Politeness motivated by the 'heart' and 'binary rationality' in Thai culture. *Journal of Pragmatics* 2012; 44: 619–35.

49 Comte-Sponville A. *A Short Treatise on the Great Virtues. The Uses of Philosophy in Everyday Life*. London: Random House; 2003.

Part II
Moving forward

6 From patient-centred to *person-centred* health care

Introduction

A 2011 editorial of the *British Medical Journal* advocated for making the twenty-first century the century of the patient.[1] This change required moving from 'the century of the doctor, the clinics, and medical industry' by producing a critical mass of informed patients and clinicians, committed to patient care.[2] The observation that 'most patients report that they are not involved or informed in decisions about their care as much as they would like to be' underpinned this vision, which a special panel had articulated to mark the signing of the 2010 Salzburg statement in support of shared decision-making.[3,4] In 2015 the *British Medical Journal* put the spotlight again on patient-centred care, this time by commissioning articles to promote increased use of patients' 'energy, insight and expertise' to strengthen patient care as 'central to the mission of healthcare'.[5]

Part I of this book, however, revealed serious limitations to the ideal of patient-centred health care and how this model has evolved and been implemented to meet policy goals for population health care. Patienthood has become a vague term detaching and incompletely describing one social role in health care. The centricity of the patient obscures the person playing this role and the implicit role of the clinician in a welfare relationship of mutual dependence. Moving health care forward therefore necessitates making more than improvements within the structure of patient-centred health care. The clinician–patient relationship itself requires reframing. So, after considering whether or not health care even needs a 'centre', this chapter explores the language of person(hood) and then the model of person-centred health care. It discusses how this latter model advances health care by constructing the clinician–patient relationship in ways that go beyond limitations inherent to patient-centredness. Person-centred health care has yet to differentiate itself clearly from patient-centred health care, but I will address this problem by outlining a generic definition of person-centred health care before Chapter 7 distinguishes person-centred health care in detailed, disaggregated terms from patient-centred health care.

The centre of health care

I have attended academic conferences where some of the delegates have challenged the need to use centrist language, such as patient-centred health care, to identify a centre of health care. The notion of a centre, they have pointed out, is ambiguous and invites questions to which answers are not easily given. What is the centre? Does it delineate what is all-important or merely most important? Is it complete? Is it fixed? Does it not implicitly marginalize moral concerns outside the centre? Why not adopt alternatives to centrist terminologies?

De-centring the concept of health care avoids the binary opposition of a centre versus margins or a periphery, and enables people to conceptualize multiple perspectives simultaneously. However, care that has no centre to cohere and stabilize it can implode. Jacques Derrida answered this concern by arguing that the centre must exist even though it must be denied and hidden. Noncentrist language can meet this need. For example, the concepts of 'goal-oriented patient care',[6] 'patient-focused care'[7] and 'patient powered healthcare',[8] 'keep patients at the implicit centre of health care; these concepts displace everything else, including clinicians, non-patients and evidence. Person-focused care'[9,10] further overcomes any privileging of patients and de-emphasizes social roles in health care. Yet none of these alternatives satisfies arguments for health care having a named centre.

The presence of such a centre provides a powerful reminder that health care, both metaphorically and literally, has a natural heart – a human, dynamic, balanced core. The ordered, muscular force of this heart keeps health care alive and vital. Making health care strong and creative, it takes health care beyond reason and evidence to what can be felt and experienced as a living, caring whole. The heart, as Blaise Pascal explained, 'has its reasons that reason knows nothing of'. It is the soul of life. Its spiritual energy extends beyond the patient to empower clinicians to assure patients (especially when their life is threatened) that they are not alone; that, as E.E. Cummings wrote, 'i carry your heart with me(i carry it in my heart)i am never without it.' For such reasons, recognizing the heart of health care appears essential. As the poet, William Butler Yeats warned in his poem, *The Second Coming*, 'without a heart the centre cannot hold; mere anarchy is loosed upon the world'.

If the heart is taken as a symbol of coherence, the 'patient' is an incomplete part of the heart – a partial, perceptual role frame, fragmented from other interdependent functions central to participation in health care. Moreover, while the patient role can overwhelm expression of the authentic person dwelling beneath it, so too is erosion of role differentiation obscuring the patient role. Equality has come to mean increasing 'sameness' rather than 'oneness', yet still the concept of patienthood cannot lose its shadow of role dependency. Drawing on William Rimmer's painting, *Flight and Pursuit* – and mindful of its inscription, 'Oh for the Horns of the Altar' – I see the patient as forced under chase to follow its shadow in vain search of a sanctuary. In summary, the patient is not a sufficient embodiment of the centre, even if it is necessarily part of the centre.

Alternative terms to describe patients include 'consumer', 'client', 'customer', 'service user' and 'enrolee'. However, besides still excluding non-patients, these terms can be more depersonalizing and objectionable to the people they are applied to than is the word, 'patient'.[11] The terms tend to commodify health care, especially when used in conjunction with other terms like 'insured lives, items on a balance sheet, or centers of profit of life ... [And likewise, clinicians are] not providers, case managers, fund holders, contractors, or mere job holders'.[12] Meanwhile, terms such as 'family- and caregiver-centred care' expand the notion of patient-centredness but are just as ambiguous. So I prefer not to redefine or completely replace the 'patient'.

Instead, I prefer to *restrict* using the word, patient, to describe a particular social role and part of social identity, without this role explicating the centre of health care. There *is* a centre, however, that includes actual and potential service users as well as service providers. Shared by patients and clinicians, the humanizing term, 'person' describes this expanded centre. It coheres the roles of different persons as well as the many roles each person plays. It also accommodates change in roles like patient and clinician without implicitly losing their constitutive value. Thus, personhood extends beyond the role of the patient to characterize the central dynamic substance of health care – with patients becoming *a* focus rather than *the* focus of this care. Only through coming to know clinicians and patients – first and foremost, as persons – can care of, and by, them respect their full moral significance by accounting for all dimensions of their personhood and relational interdependence.

Personhood

The meaning of the concept of person is itself vague, prompting ethicists such as Tom Beauchamp and James Childress[13] in their canonical text on bioethics to 'avoid it ... insofar as possible'. Yet, even though the concept is contested, it is no less unclear – and is more openly inclusive – than the concept of patient. As philosopher, Michael Loughlin[14] points out, 'in reply to the question: Should medicine care for persons or not? Few would answer in the negative'. People invoke the 'everyday meaning' of person in ordinary language, which equates to the concept of a human being. Including all patients and clinicians among others, this routine practice makes person-centred health care widely accessible as a rhetorical device of common sense. However, the habit also begs the question of the justification for equating the person and human being. To add content to this discussion of person-centredness in health care, I want to identify two conceptualizations of personhood.

1 Existential personhood

The first of these conceptualizations denotes personhood as an existential construct. Sometimes named ontological personalism, this construct signifies a state of being that, by its nature, has moral status. An individual, here, is a person not because of what the person as an individual can do or does. Rather, the attribute of personhood is evident as a quality of 'category membership'. Personhood derives from membership of a group whose biological or material attributes, including species-level capabilities, give the group – and all of its members – absolute dignity as valued ends in themselves and mandate their treatment with respect. From this perspective, every human being – as a member of the human species, *homo sapiens* – is a person. Being human, as a biological category, suffices as a condition for the individual to have the quality of personhood as a moral category. However, being human is probably not a necessary condition of personhood since one can imagine non-human beings or hybrid entities having properties that count toward personhood.

Personhood therefore is not an accessory to human existence. All humans exist as persons from the start of their life – and the roots of this anthropological conception of personhood are humanism. Being human is an embodied, biologic state with essential features amenable to empirical discovery. From a spiritual and religious perspective, existential human personhood may also unify the human body with a unique essence or soul that transcends physicality and makes this life sacred within the realm of the natural order. Critics note that life after death, except symbolically, cannot be empirically tested, and that when human life begins as well as ends is contentious. However, human life as a basis for personhood can be objectively defined in terms of the integrated function of the human being as an organism – as a form of life acting in a coordinated manner to maintain the health of the body as a whole. Medical embryology indicates that human life begins at fertilization, from which time the developing embryo is a living organism. Science further indicates that physical life ends with brain death. Coordinated bodily function ends then, even if cellular life continues for a time. Moreover, beyond the contested meaning of human life, international law recognizes all humans as persons.

From their birth in the human community, persons own – and are owed by this community – basic, inviolable and inalienable moral rights. For example, Article 6 of the United Nations General Assembly's Universal Declaration of Human Rights states that, 'Everyone has the right to recognition everywhere as a person before the law.'[15] Subsequent agreements, including the International Covenant on Economic, Social and Cultural Rights, reinforce this statement.[16] Although merely conventional, this universal declaration and its covenants on human rights, such as health (care), produce a normative impetus for implementation by signatory states.

2 Relational personhood

Personhood can also be conceived of as an emergent state characterizing the moral subjecthood and dignity of individual persons in relation to other persons. This state denotes how these persons obtain, grow or lose their own moral standing as social beings from realizing, or not, their capabilities to make and act on moral judgements within their communities. Such capabilities are constructed biologically, socially and historically from properties that describe persons as independent and interdependent beings who exhibit freedom and own opportunities for intersubjectivity and autonomy. The quality of their personal autonomy includes agency and authenticity; and so, personhood cannot be a set of tricks like that performed by Red Peter, an ape that decides to become human to escape his caged existence in Franz Kafka's short story, *A Report to an Academy*. Society defines the value of relational personhood and the rights that personhood confers.

As applied to human beings, this view of personhood draws on a long tradition. Since at least the sixth century of the Common Era, when Boethius defined a person as a subsistent individual possessing a rational nature, personhood (or full personhood) has been suggested to depend on the presence of range properties or capabilities. Over time, such properties have been mooted to include consciousness; self-awareness, incorporating the ability to feel pain; reasoning; self-concept and self-directedness; and moral attributes. A recent example of a definition of personhood from this perspective comes from Eric Cassell,[17] for whom a person is an 'embodied, purposeful, thinking, feeling, emotional, reflective, relational, human individual always in action, responsive to meaning and whose life in all spheres points both outward and inward'.

The criterial properties that define the capability to act relationally are uniformly arbitrary and difficult to validate and apply. Often they can only be inferred from intuitions and reflections on experience. Thus, some individuals, who at least sometimes cannot satisfy certain criteria, may be(come) seen as persons of a lesser kind than others, or as not persons, and not entitled to some recognized rights. A conspicuous example is how the murderer–physician, Harold Shipman, through his immoral choices, lost moral standing and some basic human freedoms. Society reconstructed his personhood for the sake of social justice. Sometimes the recalibration of personhood is based on ascribed (rather than acquired) characteristics that may be strongly contested. For example, if personhood depends on conscious experience that begins from 20 weeks gestation, then induced abortions do not violate the rights of persons. Anathema to up to 1.2 billion Catholics and 1 billion Hindus, among others around the world, this perspective has further implications for other ethical dilemmas such as the destruction of human embryonic stem cells for research purposes and therapy, and demands on health services.

3 Synthesis

Nevertheless there is scope to maximize insights from the perspectives of existential personhood *and* the relational perspective by viewing these dual perspectives not as competing but rather as answers to complementary questions. Existential personhood answers the question, 'What is a person?' with, '(At least) every human being.' This minimum standard of ontological personhood assumes that human beings have special significance on the generic basis of their distinctive nature. From this perspective, person-centred health care emphasizes that all human beings are persons. In agentic terms therefore, the centre is all encompassing. Debate about 'What is human?' and 'What is machine?' is likely, however, to become important as advances in biotechnology make human bodies increasingly dispensable and able to be manipulated and enhanced to reflect personal desires; that is, persons may ultimately become their minds. I also acknowledge that person-centredness privileges personhood above attributes such as behaviour, evidence and disease.

The question, 'Who is the person?' reconciles the existential and relational perspectives. Having recognized that every living human being is innately a person with inherent dignity and value, this question invites differentiation among individual persons. These persons can be distinguished on the basis of objective and subjective variation in their potential and realized capabilities as social beings, and their morally appropriate treatment. The question, 'Who is the person?' does not challenge their categorical equal moral status as human persons, and hence it protects some fundamental rights associated with person-hood. However, beyond that minimum protection, it recognizes that person-hood can weaken or strengthen relational bonds. The question allows for considering empirical, graded differences between persons, which can inform qualitative social judgements of changes in the nature and standing of their moral status contextually and developmentally.

Thus, whereas 'what' a person has is a shared, existential identity, 'who' the person is reflects how this identity continues to change and manifest itself differently over time and across persons in accordance with their character and capabilities. These changes shape the needs, interests and freedom of opportunity of persons to: be involved in the world; choose to do or be things they have reason to value; respond to demands they and other persons make; and flourish as persons by actualizing generic as well as individualized and diverse potentialities. This dual construction of personhood opposes actions that threaten human life and welfare, such as termination of pregnancy, while recognizing – from the earliest stages of human development – the need of persons to live good lives. Giving symbolic representation to this perspective is El Lissitzky's image, *The Constructor*. The photographer's face in the image has emerged from the shadows to see, hand-create and realize his capability for full personhood at the centre of a circle of care that doubles as a halo. The concentricity of this symbol of care reminds the viewer that care has no clear beginning or end.

Personalized medicine

While the meaning of personhood remains unresolved, interest has grown in developing a health care of the person. Personal care has long characterized clinical disciplines such as family medicine, whose practitioners seek to draw on personal knowledge of each patient, accumulated over time. They use this knowledge to inform assessments of personalized disease risks and care preferences, for example to guide screening decisions around conditions such as prostate cancer and put flesh on the bones of pre-test and post-test probabilities of serious disease. However, 'personalized medicine' goes further in focusing bio-logically on the person.

Personalized medicine reduces the person to an individual by individualizing prevention and treatment programmes. Advances in molecular medicine, genomics and bioinformatics have precipitated this development, which rede-fines the scientific evidence for medical care, implicitly to tailor this care with increasing precision to each patient. Policy initiatives such as the Precision Med-icine Institute in the United States are now growing the prospect – and for some patients the reality – of medicine taking increased account of individual variability in clinically managing cancers and ultimately a wide range of health conditions. Still uncertain, however, is how much of the risk variance in common human diseases can be accounted for, and predicted by, the human genome and be managed through gene-based drugs and other direct interven-tions. The emerging science of epigenetics is adding promise to personalized medicine. However, by definition, personalized medicine, as individualized medicine, is silent on the need to manage social determinants of population health and health inequalities, and reduces the focus on personalizing care in a holistic, relational and caring sense.

An unmet need persists for medicine and health care more generally to redis-cover patients as persons, for example through 'personomics'[18] or at least the integration of biomedical, biopsychosocial and spiritual care. Writing in the *New England Journal of Medicine* over 50 years ago, Herman Blumgart[19] warned of the risk of molecular biology curdling the milk of human kindness. His warning continues to resonate today and must be heeded because, as important as it may become, personalized medicine fails to correct for over-reliance on scientific evidence for health care decision-making, and the risk of dehumanization objec-tifying patients and subordinating clinicians' moral interests. Personalized medi-cine therefore requires an interdisciplinary and translational 'framework for science, care and management'.[20] The Evidence-Based Medicine Renaissance Group has similarly asked for evidence-based medicine to 'individualize evid-ence and share decisions through meaningful conversations in the context of a humanistic and professional clinician–patient relationship'.[21] Other leaders of evidence-based medicine answer that their model 'is fully consistent with humanistic medicine'.[22] Yet, beyond disagreement on the ability of evidence-based medicine to integrate science and humanism is the challenge that person-alized medicine poses to using epidemiologically assessed interventions, and hierarchies of evidence that privilege population data despite difficulties in gen-eralizing from them to individuals.

Humanism

It is gratifying at least to see the importance of humanistic medicine acknow-ledged. All human beings are persons. Their health care is best grounded in the human realm and more specifically in the generic origins of humanism – although not necessarily in an anthropocentrist humanism, since I have suggested that being human is merely a sufficient condition of personhood. Before reconnecting humanism to personhood in health care, I want to consider humanism itself. Humanism is a philosophical attitude or outlook, as well as a practice, ethically committed to human experience, critical thought and liberating people to find worth in their human lives. This commitment is based on moral respect for the inviolable dignity of human beings. Their value has been variously related over time to their human nature, to a divine presence in whose image humans are said to be created, to human reason and to social acceptability. The meaning of humanism today has a long history.

Traceable to ancient civilizations across the world, humanism becomes especially evident in the cosmo-centric framework of Cicero. During the High Middle Ages, humanism began to be expressed in religious terms, for example by Abu Hamid al-Ghazālī, Moses Maimonides and Thomas Aquinas. However, humanism proper emerged as a major theme during the European Renaissance, fathered by Francesco Petraca. Rediscovering classical texts, Renaissance humanism espoused the freedom of all human beings to infuse their lives actively and responsibly with *humanitas* – the ideal development of a balance of action and contemplation to achieve meaning, value, virtue and fulfilment. From about 1650 to 1800 the Enlightenment revived humanism, including a secular orientation to the natural world in the here and now, as a reaction to what was perceived as religious dogmatism. During this period the concept of relational personhood took hold through the accounts of philosophers like John Locke and Immanuel Kant. Concepts of reason, personal autonomy and moral equality established firm foundations as bases of human existence, personhood and flourishing within human communities and the non-human world. Yet it was in the mid-nineteenth and twentieth centuries that people began to identify as humanists of various types across a wide range of religious and secular contexts in and beyond Western sociologies. Resulting humanisms have included pragmatic humanism; existential humanism; and personalism, including a theistic humanism, which views persons in the relational context of a divine dynamic, and a civic and political humanism that underpins human rights law. In health care, humanistic models have been developed to emphasize the whole human experience in the clinician–patient relationship.

Humanistic models

Characteristic of humanistic models is their commitment to human caring. The concepts of care and caring are different but ambiguous and contested, as indicated in previous chapters. I view caring as a moral value and an ethical practice defining a connectedness with, and respectful and concerned attention to, concrete needs of others and oneself. As a value, caring is morally important in motivating from emotion – as well as reason – relational attendance to the needs of someone. As such, caring is both a personal disposition and a social relation that builds trust and responsiveness between persons, while carrying standards by which to evaluate its ability to meet needs. An ethics of caring relations accounts for caring experiences of the recipient of care and its provider. Health care has modelled mutuality in the caring that can take place in patient–clinician relationships.

Edmund Pellegrino and David Thomasma moved toward this position almost 30 years ago. They wrote a book that described their model of beneficence-in-trust, which mediates between paternalism and autonomy through the clinician and patient holding in trust, 'the goal of acting in the best interests of one another in the relationship'.[23] The title of the book, however, exposes that this goal is ultimately for 'The *patient's* good.' The same goal was implicit in the emerging concept of shared decision-making,[25] and in the Pew–Fetzer Taskforce[24] explicating the centrality of interpersonal relationships as a professional practice in health care and health professions education. However, in 2006, Mary Catherine Beach and Thomas Inui[26] reconstructed relationship-centred care[27] to increase attention to persons' *reciprocal* and morally valuable relationships, in which affect and emotion are key components. One argument for prioritizing the person over relationships, as Christian Smith[28] explains, is that persons are the more basic unit in ontological reality. Constitutionally they are social beings that by nature drive and depend on social relationships to live and develop; to be a person is to live relationally with others, which avoids the potential opposition between the individual and socio-relational self.

Glyn Elwyn and I[29] conceptualized health care as a 'window mirror' in the year that Beach and Inui published their paper on relationship-centred care. Similar to their model, our prototype of person-centred health care illuminates an ideal relational vision of symmetrical balance between the clinician and patient. In their interactions, these two parties can each see one another and themselves in the window mirror, a window through which they are able to view the other person opposite them but also their reflected self at the same time. This experience is like being by a window in a room in which the light on each side of the window is equally intense. Under this condition of equal luminescence, the pane of glass acts as a window and a mirror. Rendering sight as a visual metaphor for care, the model thus describes conditions under which each person can see – and care for – themselves and the other. Respecting the moral principle of equal consideration of equal moral interests, such as dignity and respect, this model effectively removes the need to choose between putting first the welfare of either the patient or the clinician in health care. Both the patient and clinician come first as persons. Hence, rather than weaken the light on the patient, the model widens the area of illumination to reveal the patient and clinician as moral equals. While relationship-centred care has developed through clinical education and population health management,[30] the metaphor of care as a window mirror has found support in disciplines such as palliative care.[31] Yet, neither of the two models has gained as much traction as its authors might have hoped.

Other, near synonyms of person-centred health care include health care that is client-centred, family-centred and woman-centred, respectively. Related models of health care that take account of the humanness of people include values-based health care;[32] narrative health care;[33] health care committed to cultural competence;[34] a casuistic approach to health care decision-making in which particulars of the case at hand guide the relative weights that clinicians assign to potential warrants for action;[45] and a phenomenological model that emphasizes everyday human experience as a practical source of the lived understanding that is needed to create personal value and meaning. Scientific understanding that evidence informs can expand this understanding in health care.[35] Similarly, whole person health care[36] focuses on humanistic care of the person as an integrated, embodied whole being who experiences their own life world. Another influential model is systems health care. It uses systems theory and informatics tools to integrate lay experts with health care professionals to answer clinically relevant questions, for example about the genome and whole human organism. To improve health outcomes, it responds to complexity and biological variability at the individual and population levels.[37] Critics of this model nevertheless question its current ability 'to conceptualize living wholes, and ... account for meaning, value and symbolic interaction'.[38] Whole person health care, by contrast, is committed to Hippocratic curing and Asklepian healing by at least one whole person in relation to another whole person.[39]

Person-centred health care

The most promising approach, given the scale and recent momentum of interest from health professionals, is person-centred health care – a model that resembles relationship-centred health care and health care as a window mirror. For a decade the World Health Organization has been championing a version of person-centred health care that it calls 'people-centred' health care, as a policy framework for reforming health care and health systems. Policies have been up-scaling people-centred care in low-income and middle-income countries.[40,41] Many high-income health systems have been similarly putting people or the person at the centre of health care; for example, England's National Health Service explicitly envisioned a 'people-centred health system' in its 2010–2015 five-year plan.[42] In turn, a person-centred ethos for health care describes the activities of professional groups such as the European Society for Person-Centred Health Care. Meanwhile the International College for Person-Centered Medicine enjoys links with professional and patient organizations like the World Medical Association, World Psychiatry Association, World Congress of Family Doctors and International Alliance of Patients' Organizations.

As noted above, most health professionals can be expected to find the term, 'person-centred health care' unobjectionable without giving much thought to its different, abstract meanings or those of the term, 'person'. These professionals, among others, are likely to apply everyday rather than theoretical understandings of person-centred health care, but they may also hold a particular view of person-centred health care or at least of what person-centred health care is *not*. They may sense that person-centred health care opposes the reductionism and scientism that critics of evidence-based medicine, in particular, have perceived to threaten clinical practice in the modern health care environment. By default, person-centred health care implies holism and practical wisdom in clinical thinking and practice. Apparent in this context is a tendency to conflate the terms 'person' and 'patient'. Other commentators distinguish between these concepts but emphasize the *patient as a person*, for example through personalized care planning for patients with long-term health conditions. I want to consider both of these fundamentally patient-centric approaches, beginning with the first one.

The National Health Service exemplifies the tendency to treat the person and the patient as semantically identical. Despite committing itself to moving toward a 'more people-centred' health system, it has implied through its commitment to 'putting patients first' that people are synonymous with patients.[43] In the United States, the Patient-Centered Outcomes Research Institute has likewise claimed to focus on people rather than patients, yet has suggested that 'decisions are made by patients ("people"), not by the physician'.[44] Similarly, the National Quality Forum recently acknowledged that, in its final report on measuring person-centred care, the terms 'individuals, persons and patients are used interchangeably'.[45] Such imprecise use of language is common and widely tolerated for other concepts in health care. An example is how the Choosing Wisely initiative continues in a growing number of health systems to focus on avoiding 'unnecessary' care when it really means 'inappropriate' care, since unnecessary care can still be appropriate and not constitute overuse.

The second body of work focuses on the patient as a person despite acknowledging the patient and clinician as persons. It defines person-centred medicine inclusively, often generically defining person-centred medicine as:

> a medicine of the person (of the totality of the person's health, including its ill and positive aspects), for the person (promoting the fulfilment of the person's life project), by the person (with clinicians extending themselves as full human beings, well grounded in science and with high ethical aspirations) and with the person (working respectfully, in collaboration and in an empowering manner through a partnership of patient, family and clinicians).[46]

This definition distinguishes the person from social roles in health care such as patient and clinician. It highlights how these different roles share the unifying attribute of the personhood of the diverse participants giving and receiving health care. Person-centred health care respects this diversity by recognizing 'the autonomy, responsibility and dignity of every person involved'.[47] Earlier in this chapter I suggested that all human beings are persons who vary in their capabilities and expression of those capabilities. It is a short step then to view person-centred health care as 'care that [for at least good human lives] recognizes and cultivates the capabilities associated with the concept of persons'.[48] In recognizing the freedom of persons to develop their capabilities in different ways, this perspective of person-centred health care makes space to recognize clinicians as persons too, and not view the 'epicentre' of health care as 'the person of the patient'. However, with a small number of exceptions,[49] authors embracing this theoretical perspective continue to focus in practice on the person of the patient and attend parenthetically to the person of the clinician, without explaining this disjuncture. By their own standards, they reduce person-centred health care to patient-centred health care.

Since patient-centred health care already recognizes the care of the patient as a whole person, the latter feature effectively locates person-centred health care within patient-centred health care.[50,51] The Gothenburg Centre for Person-Centred Care exemplifies this perspective. Work by this interdisciplinary research centre emphasizes the patient as an equal partner whose narratives contribute to a personal care plan that is developed with health care professionals, documented in the patient's record and integrated in the care process.[52] This model therefore re-dresses patient-centred health care in new linguistic clothes. It brings the personhood of the patient to the fore without distinguishing how, compared with patient-centred health care, person-centred health care signifies what the World Health Organization recognizes as a 'paradigm shift' or 'major shift in thinking'.[53] In reducing the person to the person of the patient, this practice further disregards the warning of the World Health Organization against confusing people-centred care with patient-centred care that 'comprises an important part, but not the totality, of a people-centred approach'.[54] Yet the World Health Organization itself stops short of explaining what makes the shift 'major'. Andrew Miles[55] has suggested that person-centred health care fixes the problem that patient-centred health care is fundamentally a 'patient-directed, consumerist form of care'.

Is this correct? Certainly, with the development of patient-centred health care, 'recent discourse on respect for autonomy is more explicit about promoting, supporting and being responsive to patients' autonomous choices'.[56] Patients are more involved than ever in sharing and making health care decisions, especially for highly value-laden and preference-sensitive interventions under conditions of genuine uncertainty over benefits versus harms. Also, Rule 3 of the Institute of Medicine's report, 'Crossing the Quality Chasm',[57] identifies 'the patient as the source of control.' And some commentators have advocated for the strongest form of patient autonomy in health care,[58-60] including informative[61] and patient choice models in which 'the patient makes the final choice among existing alternatives'.[62] However, besides uncertainty over who decides when there is equipoise,[63] authoritative proponents of patient-centred health care have consistently stated that patients 'are known as persons ... and their wishes are honored (but not mindlessly enacted)'.[64]

In this context, autonomous patients can accept or not the treatments offered to them by a clinician but typically, at most, patients can suggest rather than determine those treatments. Moreover, patient-centred health care, despite varied usage of this term, tends not to isolate the patient in making such decisions. It emphasizes the relational autonomy of patients, whose decisions are shared within, and because of, their care relationships with others, including clinicians. Patient autonomy is realized therefore in social circumstances in which that principle does not override other moral considerations; for example, patient-centred health care still speaks to the beneficent 'clinician-as-person' beneath the mellifluous tones of patient autonomy. For these reasons, proponents of person-centred health care need to be careful not to misrepresent patient-centred health care or equate person-centred health care with patient-centred health care. For the reasons presented in Chapter 7, patient-centred health care – even when it focuses on the 'patient-as-person' – differs from person-centred health care; and the construct of patient-as-person is insufficient to distinguish health care as person-centred.

This perspective resists the continuing focus of person-centred health care on the personhood of the patient, a focus that draws historical support from the Swiss physician, Paul Tournier[65] and other physician pioneers such as Francis Peabody.[66] Their focus on the patient as a person better describes them as progenitors of patient-centred health care than person-centred health care. The same holds true for the person-centred therapy of humanistic psychologist, Carl Rogers.[67] Closer than these models to emphasizing the personhood of the clinician and patient are: writings by the Balints, who initially described patient-centred medicine as 'whole person medicine' before deciding that it 'is rather a mouthful and much too ambitious';[68] the model of relationship-centred care;[23] work by Tom Kitwood,[69] in particular on person-centred approaches to caring for people living with dementia, and palliative care; and person-centred nursing frameworks for older people.[70-72]

The International College of Person-Centered Medicine has identified key principles of person-centred medicine,[47] but they are broad and vague. Despite the above working definition of person-centred health care, this model remains poorly understood. Thus, it seems premature at this time to implement and test models of person-centred health care, contrary to the belief that implementation should proceed 'now that earlier exercises in conceptualization have been undertaken and advanced'.[47] Without an improved understanding of person-centred health care, it makes little sense to develop operational methodologies and implement and evaluate programmes for this model. These tasks cannot properly take place until it is clear what person-centred health care signifies and how it differs from and improves on patient-centred health care.

Effectively established in 2009, the International College of Person-Centered Medicine has been less concerned with elucidating areas of similarity and difference between these models than with expressing a need 'to transform medical practice from the current disease-based, management-directed, reductionist approach'. Barbara Starfield[73] suggested that, as described in the literature, patient-centred health care has focused on visit-based care for disease management whereas person-centred health care emphasizes the accumulation over time of relational knowledge to manage patients' problems. However, this argument appears to justify a need less for person-centredness than for returning to founding principles of patient-centred health care, such as longitudinality of care. Rachel Davis and I have suggested that the moral equality of persons is a value distinguishing person-centred health care from patient-centred health care's basic principle of primacy of patient welfare. Person-centred health care meets a need, unmet by patient-centred health care, to explicate how equal moral interests of patients and clinicians, as persons, interconnect to balance and maximize their joint welfare. Yet, a comprehensive framework is still needed for conceptualizing person-centred health care.

As Leonardo da Vinci pointed out over a half a millennium ago, 'he who loves practice without theory is like the sailor who boards ship without a rudder and compass and never knows where he may cast'. And as the philosopher, George Santayana reminded the world, in discussing how knowledge is acquired, there is a risk of mistakes from history repeating themselves if their lessons are not learnt. The multiple reconstitutions of evidence-based medicine[74] exemplify the dangers of waiting nearly two decades to publish a clear explication of this model's epistemic assumptions.[75] And so, to close this chapter, I want to provide a short, generic definition of person-centred health care as a *value-strong ethic of virtue*. The next chapter will disaggregate this definition into values of person-centred health care that support the cultivation and exercise of virtue by clinicians and patients. It will compare these values with those of patient-centred health care as a *duty-based ethic* that: puts patient welfare first and respects patient autonomy and social justice; does not obligate praiseworthy motives of clinicians; and is generally quiet on patient responsibilities and clinician welfare.

Generic model

Person-centred health care puts persons first. Contemporary moral and political philosophy generally acknowledges that all persons are moral equals in some sense. From this premise of basic equality, patients and clinicians count equally as human persons *sui generis* who share fundamentally equal moral interests even within their inherently unequal relationship. The equality of these interests, such as to treatment with respect, warrants their equal consideration. No weakening of patient welfare is implied. To the contrary, *adding* the person of the clinician to the centre of health care illuminates and dignifies the welfare of the person of the patient as well as of the clinician, whose welfare is integrally connected to the welfare of the patient. No scarcity of welfare is role-distributed on a hierarchical basis like need. Each person can be(come) their best self – and hence everyone 'wins' when clinicians and patients realize their capability to care for each other and themselves in mutually beneficial ways responsive to each party's equal and interdependent moral interests.

Such caring depends less on a set of abstract moral principles for patient welfare than on the prior development and exercise of good character by clinicians and patients. Good, stable character, or virtue, is needed because it can be trusted to produce consistently and situationally good cooperative behaviour faithful to the sense that persons have of who they are and want to strive to become. Grounded in deeply held values, good character disposes persons to put their moral values relationally into practice. The next chapter, as noted above, will discuss these values. They commit clinicians and patients to trust each other joyfully to reciprocate care, according to their equal moral interests within the limits of their capabilities. The goal here is to try to construct balanced win-win decisions that, without requiring compromise on either side, fully satisfy each party and enable the patient and clinician to flourish. As such, person-centred health synthesizes the sciences and humanities to nourish capabilities of patients and clinicians to thrive in their interdependency and lead good lives. Readers may wonder what this model does to altruism, as the 'essence of professionalism'.[76]

Some disciplines – most notably, evolutionary biology and economics – have challenged the notion of altruism. However, altruism can be understood in different ways. Person-centred health care, as I have constructed it, can accommodate altruism that is defined as 'taking the interests of the other as one's own'.[77] This definition keeps intact the self and other. In contrast, I have long struggled with definitions that dissolve the self through describing altruism as selfless giving whose purpose is to promote the interests only of the other. In common with Aristotle I prefer to retain but integrate the distinction between self and other and recognize how even self-sacrifice can be responsive to self-interest and felt duty. For example, the health care workers who manage highly infectious outbreaks, such as Ebola, act with safe courage to do what their conscience tells them must be done. Otherwise they deny their internal morality and put themselves and others at risk of harm. Altruism here retains 'fidelity to the self', in the words of the philosopher, Michel Terestchenko.[78]

Conclusion

In response to serious limitations of patient-centred health care, this chapter has introduced concepts relating to personhood and the model of person-centred health care. I have indicated my preference for using the concept of existential personhood to identify all human beings as persons. At the same time, insights from relational personhood indicate the social standing, needs and opportunities of persons to nurture or squander their capabilities for full personhood. Person-centred health care transitions between these complementary concepts of personhood by building capabilities for flourishing and leading a good life. For person-centred health care to continue to develop, however, writers and practitioners will need explicitly to define – and as far as possible reach agreement on – what they mean by personhood and how, in health care, this meaning and its implications differ from, and can be preferred to, the nomenclature of patienthood. Distinguishing person-centred health care from personalized medicine, I have sketched how person-centred health care has come to be understood in the context of its historical evolution and current usage. But I have also progressed the task of distinguishing it from patient-centred health care by suggesting an inclusive generic definition of person-centred health care. Chapter 7 details how modest foundational values of person-centred health care can sustain a virtue ethic that differs from, and advances, values of patient-centred health. At least implicitly, these values nourish the personal care needs that Part I revealed from clinician to patient, clinician to self, patient to self, and patient to clinician.

References

1 Gulland A. Welcome to the century of the patient. *British Medical Journal* 2011; 342: d2057.

2 Gigerenzer G, Muir Gray JA. Launching the century of the patient. In: Gigerenzer G, Muir Gray JA, editors. *Better Doctors, Better Patients, Better Decisions: Envisioning Health Care 2020.* Cambridge, MA: Massachusetts Institute of Technology and the Frankfurt Institute for Advanced Studies 2011; pp. 3–28.

3 *Salzburg Global Seminar. The Salzburg statement on shared decision making.* 2011; http://e-patients.net/u/2011/03/Salzburg-Statement.pdf.

4 Nageshwaran S, Choudhury M, Nageshwaran S. 'Patient-centredness' and 'Shared decision making' are inextricably linked. *British Medical Journal* 2011; 342: d2117.

5 Richards T, Coulter A, Wicks P. Time to deliver patient centred care. *British Medical Journal* 2015; 350.

6 Reuben D, Tinetti M. Goal-oriented patient care – an alternative health outcomes paradigm. *New England Journal of Medicine* 2012; 366: 777–9.

7 Walker JEC. Concepts of patient care for the 1960's. *Bulletin of the New York Academy of Medicine* 1965; 41: 118–24.

8 deBronkart D. From patient centred to people powered: autonomy on the rise. *British Medical Journal* 2015; 350.

9 Starfield B. Is Patient-Centered Care the same as Person-Focused Care? *Permanente Journal* 2011; 15: 63–9.

10 Fraser J. Comforts of home: home care of the terminally ill. *Canadian Family Physician.* 1990; 36: 977–81.

11 Deber R, Kraetschmer N, Urowitz S, Sharpe N. Patient, consumer, client, or customer: what do people want to be called? *Health Expectations* 2005; 8: 345–51.

12 Pellegrino ED. Medical ethics in an era of bioethics: resetting the medical profession's compass. *Theoretical Medicine and Bioethics* 2012; 33: 21–4.

13 Beauchamp TL, Childress JF. *Principles of Biomedical Ethics.* Sixth edition. Oxford: Oxford University Press; 2009.

14 Loughlin M. What person-centered medicine is and isn't: temptations for the 'soul' of PCM. *European Journal for Person-Centered Healthcare* 2014; 2: 16–21.

15 United Nations General Assembly. Universal Declaration of Human Rights. 1948; 217 A (III).

16 United Nations. International Covenant on Economic, Social and Cultural Rights. New York: United Nations; 1966.

17 Cassell E. The person in medicine. *International Journal of Integrated Care* 2010; 10: 50–2.

18 Ziegelstein R. Personomics. *JAMA Internal Medicine* 2015; 175: 888–9.

19 Blumgart HL. Caring for the patient. *New England Journal of Medicine* 1964; 270: 449–56.

20 Evers A, Rovers M, Kremer J, Veltman J, Schalken J, Bloem B, van Gool A. An integrated framework of personalized medicine: from individual genomes to participatory health care. *Croatian Medical Journal* 2012; 53: 301–3.

21 Greenhalgh T, Howick J, Maskrey N, Evidence Based Medicine Renaissance Group. Evidence-based medicine: a movement in crisis? *British Medical Journal* 2014; 348: g3725.

22 Post PN, Guyatt GH. Evidence-based medicine offers an optimal starting point for person-centered medicine. *European Journal for Person Centered Healthcare* 2014; 2: 76–8.

23 Pellegrino ED, Thomasma DC. *For the Patient's Good: The Restoration of Beneficence in Health Care*. New York: Oxford University Press; 1988.

24 C. P. Tresolini and The Pew-Fetzer Task Force. Health Professions Education and Relationship-centered Care. San Francisco, CA: Pew Health Professions Commission; 1994.

25 President's Commission for the Study of Ethical Problems in Medicine and Biomedical and Behavioral Research. Making health care decisions. The ethical and legal implications of informed consent in the patient–practitioner relationship. Washington DC: US Government Printing Office; 1982.

26 Beach M, Inui T, Relationship-Centered Care Research Network. Relationship-centered care: a constructive reframing. *Journal of General Internal Medicine* 2006; 21: S3–8.

27 Magee M. Relationship-based health care in the United States, United Kingdom, Canada, Germany, South Africa and Japan. World Medical Association Assembly; Finland. 2003 (11 September).

28 Smith C. *To Flourish or Destruct*. Chicago: University of Chicago Press; 2015.

29 Buetow S, Elwyn G. The window mirror: a new model of the patient–physician relationship. *Open Medicine* 2008; 2: E20–25.

30 Nundy S, Oswald J. Relationship-centered care: a new paradigm for population health management. *Healthcare* 2014; 2: 216–19.

31 Janssen A, MacLeod R. Who cares for whom? Reciprocity of care at the end of life. *Journal of Palliative Care and Medicine* 2012; 2: 129.

32 Fulford KWM. *Moral Theory and Medical Practice*. Cambridge: Cambridge University Press; 1989.

33 Greenhalgh T. Narrative based medicine in an evidence based world. *British Medical Journal* 1999; 318: 323–5.

34 Betancourt J, Green A, Carrillo E, Park E. Cultural competence and health care disparities: key perspectives and trends. *Health Affairs* 2005; 24: 499–505.

35 Schwartz MA, Wiggins O. Science, humanism and the nature of medical practice: a phenomenological view. *Perspectives in Biology and Medicine* 1985; 28: 331–61.

36 Hutchinson T, editor. *Whole Person Care. A New Paradigm for the 21st Century*. New York: Springer; 2011.

37 Noble D. *The Music of Life: Biology beyond the Genome*. Oxford: Oxford University Press; 2006.

38 Vogt H, Ulvestad E, Polit T, Getz L. Getting personal: can systems medicine integrate scientific and humanistic conceptions of the patient? *Journal of Evaluation in Clinical Practice* 2014; 20: 942–52.

39 Hutchinson T, editor. *Whole Person Care. A New Paradigm for the 21st Century*. New York: Springer; 2011.

40 World Health Organization (WHO). People-centred care in low- and middle-income countries. Geneva: WHO; 2010.

41 Rathi A, Jilani A, Trivedi J. Making health care more person-centred in low and middle income countries: a consideration of possible strategies with an emphasis on south-east Asia. *International Journal of Person Centered Medicine* 2011; 1: 463–7.

42 NHS England. NHS 2010–2015: from good to great: preventative, people-centred, productive. Redditch: Department of Health; 2009.

43 NHS England. Putting patients first. The NHS England business plan for 2013/14–2015/16. Redditch: NHS England; 2013.

44 Patient-Centered Outcomes Research Institute (PCORI). Patient-Centered Outcomes Research Definition Revision. Response to Public Input. Consensus definition as of 15 February 2012. Washington DC: PCORI; 2012.

45 National Quality Forum. Priority setting for healthcare performance measurement: addressing performance measure gaps in person-centered care and outcomes. Final Report. Washington DC: National Quality Forum; 2014.

46 Miles A, Mezzich J. Advancing the global communication of scholarship and research for personalized healthcare. *International Journal of Person Centered Medicine* 2011; 1: 1–5.

47 Miles A, Mezzich J. The care of the patient and the soul of the clinic: person centered medicine as an emergent model of modern clinical practice. *International Journal of Person Centered Medicine* 2011; 1: 207–22.

48 Entwistle V, Watt I. Treating patients as persons: using a capabilities approach to support delivery of person-centred care. *American Journal of Bioethics* 2013; 13: 29–39.

49 Rüedi B. Retaining the person in medical science. In: Cox J, Campbell A, Fulford KWM, editors. *Medicine of the Person. Faith, Science and Values in Health Care Provision.* London: Jessica Kingsley 2007; pp. 46–55.

50 Tanenbaum S. What is patient-centered care? A typology of models and missions. *Health Care Analysis* 2015; 23: 272–87.

51 Olsson L-E, Karlsson J, Berg J, Kärrholm J, Hansson E. Person-centred care compared with standardized care for patients undergoing total hip arthroplasty – a quasi-experimental study. *Journal of Orthopaedic Surgery and Research* 2014; 9: 95.

52 Ekman I. *Personcentrering inom hälso – och sjukvård. Fran filosofi till praktik.* Stockholm: Liber; 2013.

53 World Health Organization. What is people-centred health care? Patient at the Centre of Care Initiative. Geneva: WHO Regional Office for the Western Pacific; 2006.

54 World Health Organization (WHO). People at the centre of health care: harmonising mind and body, people and systems. Geneva: WHO; 2007.

55 Miles A. Science, humanism, judgement, ethics: person-centered medicine as an emergent model of modern clinical practice. *Folia Medicine (Plovdiv)* 2013; 55: 5–24.

56 Ellis C, Hunt MR, Chambers-Evans J. Relational autonomy as an essential component of patient-centred care. *International Journal of Feminist Approaches to Bioethics* 2011; 4: 79–101.

57 Institute of Medicine. *Crossing the Quality Chasm: A New Health System for the 21st Century.* Washington DC: National Academy Press; 2001.

58 Veatch R. *Patient, Heal Thyself. How the 'New Medicine' Puts the Patient in Charge.* Oxford: Oxford University Press; 2008.

59 McNutt R. Shared medical decision making. Problems, process, progress. *Journal of the American Medical Association* 2004; 292: 2516–18.

60 Berwick D. What 'patient-centered' should mean: confessions of an extremist. *Health Affairs* 2009; 28: w555–w565.

61 Emanuel EJ, Emanuel L. Four models of the physician–patient relationship. *Journal of the American Medical Association* 1992; 267: 2221–6.

62 Sandman L, Munthe C. Shared decision making, paternalism and patient choice. *Health Care Analysis.* 2010; 18: 60–84.

63 Wyer P, Silva SA, Post S, Quinlan P. Relationship-centred care: antidote, guidepost or blind alley? The epistemology of 21st century health care. *Journal of Evaluation in Clinical Practice* 2014; 20: 881–9.

64 Epstein R, Street Jr. R. The values and value of patient-centered care. *Annals of Family Medicine* 2011; 9: 100–3.

65 Tournier P. *Medicine de la Personne.* Neufchatel: Delachaux et Niestle; 1940.

66 Peabody F. The care of the patient. *Journal of the American Medical Association* 1927; 88: 877.

67 Rogers C. *A Way of Being.* Boston: Houghton Mifflin; 1980.

68 Balint M, Ball DH, Hare ML. Training medical students in patient-centred medicine. *Comprehensive Psychiatry* 1969; 10: 249–58.

69 Kitwood T. *Dementia Reconsidered: The Person Comes First.* Buckingham: Open University Press; 1997.

70 McCormack B. A conceptual framework for person-centred practice with older people. *International Journal of Nursing Practice* 2003; 9: 202–9.

71 Nolan M, Davies S, Brown J, Keady J, Nolan J. Beyond 'person-centred' care: a new vision for gerontological nursing. *International Journal of Older People Nursing* 2004; 13: 45–53.

72 McCormack B, McCance T. *Person-Centred Nursing: Theory and Practice.* Oxford: Wiley-Blackwell; 2010.

73 Starfield B. Is patient-centered care the same as person-focused care? *Permanente Journal* 2011; 15: 63–9.

74 Charles C, Gafni A, Freeman E. The evidence-based medicine model of clinical practice: scientific teaching or belief-based preaching? *Journal of Evaluation in Clinical Practice* 2011; 17: 597–605.

75 Djulbegovic B, Guyatt G. Epistemologic inquiries in evidence-based medicine. *Cancer Control* 2009; 16: 158–68.

76 American Board of Internal Medicine. *Project Professionalism.* Philadelphia: American Board of Internal Medicine; 1998.

77 Scott N, Seglow J. *Altruism.* Berkshire: Open University Press; 2008.

78 Terestchenko M. *Un si fragile vernis d'humanité: Banalité du mal, banalité du bien.* Paris: Découverte; 2007.

7 Person-centred health care
Values and virtues

Introduction

Person-centred health care is a values-based ethic of virtue that emphasizes developing the good character of the clinician and patient as *persons first* in order to realize their interdependent capabilities to flourish. This chapter discusses how the clinician and patient can cultivate and exercise good character and virtues from identifying with fundamental values of person-centred health care. To this end, the chapter distinguishes these values individually from corresponding values of patient-centred health care and compares the values where they differ. The rationale for this analysis is to describe and understand each of the two model's value structure, and how it is organized and functions, in order to facilitate differentiation between them. Complementing the generic definitions suggested for each model in previous chapters, this disaggregated approach anatomizes patient-centred health care and person-centred health care. Just as deconstructed food dishes have separately arranged components, these models are shown to be overlapping but distinctive entities whose multiple discrete dimensions fit together. Although these individual dimensions provide only a partial view, jointly they compose a comprehensive portrait of health care that is more vivid and detailed than generic descriptions can create.

From values to virtues

All health care is laden with values, which describe what people freely and fundamentally care about. More specifically, values are defined here as preferred endpoints of questions asking people to justify what they care about – to explain what makes them confident in their caring.[1] As Miles Little has explained, there is a 'need to ask more questions, to repeat the "*Why?*" until there is no further answer, because we have reached the level beyond which we cannot reason. That level is the level of our *values*'.[2] It follows that reasoned values yield beliefs about how things *are*. People, regardless of what they want, may value giving service, for example, because that is how their society functions. Their values may be assumed or spelt out in such general terms that no one questions them. Making values explicit can help people to understand why they hold particular preferences, but values are not preferences and are morally neutral beyond their social recognition as 'irreducible goods that humans universally accept as components of an acceptable life'.[3] Values in these terms are descriptive rather than prescriptive. They signify beliefs that may be moral. Virtues are the values selected and refined as *necessary for moral living*, for example on the basis of religious beliefs or social consensus.

Virtues are needed because, contrary to scholars like Kenneth Fulford,[4] values cannot suffice as analytical constructs whose balancing can help to make directly action-guiding moral judgements from facts. Virtues of moral agents add the guidance required to understand and evaluate the relative moral standing of different values in particular situations, and then make and enact moral decisions that bridge the gap between these values and real life. Contemporary physician groups illustrate this unmet need for virtue. The American College of Physicians[5] has identified and responded to threatened core values, such as professionalism and respect, by (re)stating moral principles and commitments for professional behaviour. Yet this leap from values to principles discounts how physicians interpret the meaning of values and move from this meaning to realize moral norms.

For example, the principle of primacy of patient welfare contradicts and trumps the value that the American College of Physicians has attached to respect for 'every human being'.[5] This disjuncture may be avoided or at least given increased transparency by constructing a virtue such as justice from its root value of equal respect. Note how the virtue of justice adds moral information. It elucidates how well or not the moral principle of primacy of patient welfare fits the value of equal respect. Here the fit feels strained because privileging patients is a form of positive discrimination, which is still discrimination and, I have been suggesting, non-functional and unjust. Person-centred health care highlights the need and opportunity to derive virtues from values to create a moral language that mediates the move from values to principled action. In this context, values remain necessary despite their insufficiency, for example in evaluating facts to support moral decision-making.

In models such as person-centred health care, persons share values that are modestly foundational in nature and importance because, 'without some foundational values to underpin the status claimed by personhood, the arguments for person-centred medicine are incomplete'.[6] Following Little, the values give basic coherence to social practices. Some writers[7] contend that person-centred health care requires no such epistemic base to support it and 'can operate well within a dynamic emergent framework'. However, a base or centre does not preclude such a framework. The values in which health care is rooted – and which frequently are hidden – give form to what grows from them. External forces can disrupt this natural growth and sprout new growth. Yet, needing only to be justifiable, values embedded as modest foundations allow subsequent regeneration to take place. Deep roots insulate the values from challenge even though future knowledge may eventually strengthen them. Even if particular values, such as personalism, are immutable, their meaning and significance may vary within and between persons over time and place. Little and his colleagues[3] have identified three foundational values of health care: survival, security and flourishing. The International Charter for Human Values in Healthcare has similarly identified core values for physicians and educators.[8] However, the values I wish to identify and discuss are those distinguishing person-centred health care from patient-centred health care.

Table 7.1 contrasts values associated respectively with each of these two models. Constructed for heuristic purposes, the value binaries are less rigid and clearly demarcated than they may appear. My seven values of person-centred health care are: flourishing, virtue, personalism, equality, pæanism, authenticity and consilience. Corresponding values are noted for patient-centred health care. Clinicians and patients share the values of the care model within which they operate even though, within their own moral space, clinicians and patients may apply the values in role-specific ways. As a value-based virtue ethic, person-centred health care moves from values to virtues to show how moral agents put moral flesh on the bones of their values. The virtues, as noted above, are always moral, derive their value from this morality, and use that value to provide a moral check on how persons apply their own values. One of these values is, itself, virtue, which supports prudence. There is no intention in the table to limit the individual virtues to their illustrative, ancestral values.

As selected moral values, the virtues describe context-sensitive strengths and practices of good character, which are expressed in response to, and are robust within, everyday situations. By character I mean stable, patterned traits of personality acquired through practice. Good traits characterize moral persons, who are disposed and energized to live fully. Thus, the virtues go beyond the strength of will that persons may have in order to act from a motive of duty, since 'Duties and obligations make sense not in themselves, but in relation to the idea of living most fully ... they are not to be seen as definitive of virtue.'[9] The virtues dispose persons to do what a person with the relevant virtues and capabilities would do in the circumstances at hand, and why, which acts against the possibility of circumstances per se determining their behaviour. In turn, the virtues progressively enable persons to realize their capabilities to flourish every day and live moral lives of excellence.

I need here to explain both what I do not mean by moral excellence and what I do mean. What I do not mean is moral saintliness or even righteousness that restricts rather than enables personal behaviour – although there cannot be an excess of virtue. The clinician and patient of virtue need not, therefore, be extraordinary persons. Nor must they be inspirational, heroic or ideal embodiments of others like them, or even evince moral excellence by being 'persons with a limited repertoire of exceptional virtues'.[10] Nevertheless, such special persons exist and virtue is not mundane. It describes persons whose prospering vocation is to be(come) the best they can be in any given place and time in order to live fully as moral beings. Returning to their deep values, they strive to know and appreciate with faith, humility and compassion the power and limitations of themselves and others as authentic beings who celebrate and honour

Table 7.1 Comparing person-centred and patient-centred health care

Person in person-centred health care	Virtue	Self-actualization	Prudence	Humanity	Justice	Fidelity	Caring	Humour	Good faith	Interdependence
Person-centred health care	Value	Flourishing	Virtue	Personalism	Moral equality	Mutual trust	Reciprocated care	Paenism	Authenticity	Consilience
Patient-centred health care	Health		Duty	Role theory	Patient welfare	Patient autonomy	Patient care	Self-control	Emotion management	Service

human life. They also have vices they manage prudently, because still relevant today is Abraham Lincoln's observation that, 'It has been my experience that folks who have no vices have very few virtues.' Thus, despite the moral giants whose actions may indicate the power of moral choice,[11] most people have mixed character traits – without which their virtues lack meaning. Only by knowing how these people manage their vices can their true measure as persons be properly assessed.

As conceptualized by Aristotle's Doctrine of the Golden Mean, persons exercise virtues that signify a desirable and feasible middle path between excess and deficiency, whose discernment through careful judgement is relative to the particulars of the situation at hand and the person. For example, straddling cowardice and recklessness is courage which, by nature, is a virtue and operates as a virtue when exercised in good pursuits. Courage enables the person to overcome their fear without going too far or not far enough. This truth is universal. The same moderation and balance that allow the person to master their circumstances, for example, infuse the Hindu text, Bhagavad Gita and the Confucian Doctrine of the Mean. Similarly, the Taoist perspective is that the person of true virtue has virtue-relevant and accessible goals that, forming a stable part of their character, motivate them to behave in a manner that is unselfconsciously, unobtrusively and unaffectedly virtuous. This person lives in harmony with life for its own sake; that is, as its own intrinsic reward. Knowing the limits of their place in the world, they eschew hubris, for example in relation to scientific prowess. They act not for approval from others but from the natural energy of humble self-appreciation that nurtures their learnt sense of what is good and lends itself to harmony. This perspective puts the virtues within reach, as moderately demanding goals.

Under material and social–structural conditions conducive to personal flourishing, persons acquire virtues by practising them frequently, and for the right reasons across different types of familiar situations, so that they become automatic and routine. Skilled in the natural art of living acquired through experience of different situations and from practice, virtuous persons therefore strive to move for the most part beyond controlled and intentional cognitive processes, such as deliberation through rational thinking. They learn to apply heuristics habitually to patterns they have recognized from memory in relevant situations, and flourish. Yet, 'Until recently, the language of virtue and the importance of virtue-based behaviour have been neglected.'[12]

Current (re)vitalization of person-centred health care coincides with the recent development of an extensive and growing literature on the virtues. This chapter will draw on literature that tends to focus on the 'virtuous clinician'[13–15] for the sake of clinician self-care and because, as the Renaissance physician, Paracelsus observed, 'The character of the physician may act more powerfully upon the patient than the drugs employed.' However, a focus on virtue and good character applies also to patients. The 'virtuous patient'[16] complements the 'expert' patient, the patient who has become 'expert' at living with, and self-managing, their long-term condition(s). From developing virtue, clinicians and patients can care for themselves and each other, specifically through the care that can take place from clinician to patient, patient to self, clinician to self and patient to clinician. In this context I will focus on the shared nature of the virtues to which clinicians and patients, as persons, may strive.

In recognizing the virtues as universally necessary for clinicians and patients to unify their good character and social roles, this approach resists the notion of role-constituted virtues.[17] It is the form or practical exercise of role-independent virtues that varies for each person in response to social roles, other circumstances and critique from outside the roles. Alasdair MacIntyre[18] pointed out that some of the virtues differ between societies and, over time, generate what Robert Veatch[19] described as 'the chaos of lists of virtues' for moral living and health care. However, empirical research suggests a generally more settled picture[20] and, beyond my example of courage, moral rules are no more immune than the virtues to philosophical objections. In this context, the core virtues appear to include prudence and courage among clinicians and patients,[13,21] as well as justice, temperance and humanity.[20] These virtues yield an ethical system that, in contrast to codes like the Physician Charter, clinicians and patients may endorse from reason, experience and secular and religious perspectives.

Overall then, my discussion constructs person-centred health care on the basis of deep values as modest foundations that resource persons to develop virtues and live fully. I will discuss, in turn, each of the seven values of person-centred health care shown in Table 7.1. This approach will reflect my personal perspective, informed by experience and literature drawn from diverse disciplines. I will compare each value to a corresponding value of patient-centred health care, and link each identified value of person-centred health care to one or more virtues of clinicians and patients. Intended to be comprehensive, the table subsumes under these different values the values common to both models. This positioning of person-centred health care, as a value-based ethic of virtue, is overdue. However, before comparing person-centred health care and patient-centred health care, I should reiterate that the latter model – in common with evidence-based medicine until quite recently[22,23] and in contrast to relationship-centred health care[24] – has weakly explicated its own assumptions.

Proponents of patient-centred health care have explained why they prefer their model to clinician-centred health care but their model has never been consistently conceptualized. They have largely taken for granted that the primacy of patient welfare is a fundamentally important moral principle guiding the care that health professionals provide. Ronald Epstein[25] has suggested that patient-centred health care reflects 'deep respect for patients as unique living beings, and the obligation to care for them on their terms' – but why, exclusively, patients? What gives patient-centred health care epistemological and moral priority as a model of health care? Underlying confusion about the meaning of patient-centred care requires my discussion of the values of this model, like those of person-centred health care, to draw on my personal reading of each model.

Joint flourishing

Patient-centred health care and person-centred health care appear similar in their commitment to strengthen health care delivery. However, the purpose of each model differs subtly in its outcomes focus. In emphasizing benevolence, patient-centred health care commits to buttressing patient health and welfare. Welfare is larger than health, which patient-centred health care tends to construct as an objective state of being well, as exemplified by an absence of disease; as an evaluative state, describing, for example, persons who perceive themselves as ill; or both, as in the World Health Organization's 1948 definition of human health as 'a state of complete physical, mental and social well-being and not merely the absence of disease or infirmity'. Most criticism of this last definition has centred on the word 'complete' but the meaning of 'well-being' is also contested. I want to suggest that health and welfare are less states of being than signifiers of becoming.

Health and welfare signify this temporal potential to 'become other' than one is – for persons to understand and redefine who they are by projecting forward into possibilities for themselves, while bringing their past with them. Redolent of the concept of the process of 'arche-health,'[26] this personal reality of, and commitment to, continuing transformation and growth resists constructing health as a stable, unifying identity. Person-centred health care further echoes this resistance by accounting for the shifting welfare of patients and clinicians in terms of striving for a positive becoming or flourishing within interrelated and complex life projects.

In these dynamic, overlapping projects, patients and clinicians can cooperate to grow and form as persons. Through cooperating they can learn not only to know things but also inwardly to become persons capable of producing integrative 'win-win' agreements. Bridging their respective positions, such agreements help them to realize their shared moral values and relational capabilities to live a good life. This life is a mutually dependent and balanced life of virtue, disposing them to live in the present but continuously learn from the past. From a Māori perspective, the past is not behind them, as in the Western sequencing of time. Rather, they can look forward through the filter of past experience and knowledge towards the future. Their commitment is to learn to experience their personhood fully. Thus, despite a rising number of studies associating health with desirable personal characteristics and a moral lifestyle, this vision of welfare in terms of becoming and self-actualization goes beyond living healthily in the now. It signifies a life in which patients and clinicians develop and exercise their joint capabilities to care richly for themselves and each other. Clinicians and patients flourish when patients care about themselves and their clinician, and clinicians self-care and care for patients. In contrast to Christian Smith, however, I do not view flourishing as a project necessarily requiring a lifetime to express personhood fully.

Flourishing may be evident episodically at particular moments in time even if not also as a way of life and over the course of a lifetime. Flourishing has more to do with the journey to become virtuous[27] and with the person making valued, dispositional progress toward realizing this aspirational state than in necessarily fully reaching it as an ultimate destination. For Smith, existential experience of personal flourishing progressively develops and actualizes the basic human goods and interests collectively required for flourishing. However, I contend that together these goods are not always necessary for flourishing. Individually, they energize and facilitate flourishing, but flourishing does not hinge on well-being as a condition of becoming, and hence can take place in its absence even at the end of life. Flourishing then depends on how the person *responds* to the spectre and reality of illness and death. As Smith acknowledges, ontologically persons are able to flourish relative to their opportunities to realize their capabilities to learn and practise virtue. These opportunities are shaped by, and shape, personal, social–structural and environmental conditions conducive, and not harmful, to flourishing.

Virtue

Patient-centred health care is, above all, deontological. It assumes that general norms of a common morality find codified and impartial expression in fundamental principles, duties and rights. These norms are assumed to transcend situational variation and differences in values and perspectives across health care practice; in respect of how known and unknown limitations of human knowledge produce unpredictability and uncertainty.[28] This ethic is apparent from patient-centric codifications of physician behaviour like the Physician Charter, which commits physicians – on the basis of professional duty – to adhere to ethical principles like primacy of patient welfare and respect for patient autonomy. Adherence to these principles and to commitments derived from them is congruent with rational application of the patient-centred clinical method, including elicitation and shared understanding of, and respect for, patients' values, concerns and preferences. Respect for patient autonomy, for example, underpins clinicians' duty to empower patients to participate in health care decision-making.

One implication is that persons cannot be characterized as having virtues, such as respectfulness, without adhering consistently to such logically *prior* moral principle(s). It would then follow that the virtues dispose these persons to be sensitive to, and act in accord with, these foundational, reasoned principles that codify necessary and sufficient conditions of goodness. However, I wish to challenge this belief. To assume that virtues derive purposefully from principles invites questions about the values and character of the moral agents from whose functioning the principles have developed; assumes that a set of principles can suffice to capture moral knowledge; restricts the role of virtue and invites the belief that, as a motivational framework, virtue lacks the moral force of principles and duties.[29] Therefore, I wish to suggest that virtues precede principles.

Moral principles, while necessary to help manage the moral shortcomings and behaviour of non-virtuous persons, *presuppose* values and virtues. The principle of considering equal interests, for example, is not epistemologically prior to the virtue of justice. Rather the principle is shaped by, and codifies, the value of moral equality and the virtue of justice. Otherwise, principles such as patient participation can act against the spirit of virtues like gratitude and foster a sense of entitlement that hinders relationship building. General, abstract principles, duties and rights can be inadequate without foundational virtues to guide their construction and application, and cannot even adequately express some virtues such as courage because moral life is frequently complex, ambiguous and non-codifiable. 'Humanity is not [fully] captured in common denominators.'[30] Removed from the milieu of moral choices in everyday health care, abstract moral principles lack enough information about the contingencies, particularities and motivational structures of individual encounters.

Principles or reasoned arguments that appear incomplete also enlarge the need for exceptions and caveats. Of course, most moral norms have exceptions, which can be separately managed and are not sufficient cause for rejection.[28] Moreover, exceptions do not refute principles whose key purpose is to change the world rather than reflect it. However, this qualification does not rescue principles such as primacy of patient welfare, to which many appropriate exceptions cast doubt on whether moral judgements need to appeal to such principles. This perspective undermines the sufficiency of connecting moral practice and principles. The ground of morality is not principles but rather a shared understanding of values and virtues of persons in their particular situation.

I am constructing person-centred health care therefore as a virtue–ethical approach that defines right action from appeal to moral values and, in turn, good character in the context of a well-lived life. Within person-centred clinical encounters, this approach offers clinicians and patients at least three key sets of related benefits. First, it moves care of the person beyond the impersonalism, directedness and incompleteness that can otherwise characterize normative principles. It also resists the argument that situations rather than character traits determine personal behaviour. By taking a middle path between these two poles of influence, it allows virtues to interact with situations in ways that take moral account of the complex particularity of local factors. This account generates context-sensitive reasons for acting from ways of moral being within narrow social spaces.

Second, although the same person may exercise particular virtues in some situations but not others, the virtues: are considered *universalist* to the extent that persons may imagine moral reasons for decisions with which they disagree; but have a *generalist* strain since, as noted above, particulars such as social roles are not epistemologically prior to values and virtues; and provide a *stable* structure motivating persons to live a good life, whatever their circumstances. Only certain situations, such as extraordinary ones, tend to weaken the predictability of character's influence. Indeed, loss of virtue can only be inferred from how persons act; truly virtuous persons are rare;[31] and when exercised freely and purposefully *within* specific situations, robust virtues act against the schizophrenia that can result from making duty the motivation for moral behaviour.

Third, a person-centred ethic of virtue remedies the failure of statements like the Physician Charter to say much about the interests, values and virtues that clinicians need in practice. These needs include their self-care and management of both increasingly complex ethical dilemmas – for example around appropriate use of medical technologies – and unintended variation in clinical care. Contextualized and particularistic management of this variation facilitates best use of the current principles in a free, spontaneous and habitual manner.

Personalism

Recognizing the reality and unique dignity of persons, person-centred health care puts persons first, not patients first. From reason, experience or even revelation, it puts persons and their lives and relationships – that is, the moral philosophy of *personalism* – explicitly at the heart of health care theory and practice. Personalism takes many different forms including, since at least the late nineteenth century, American personalism and then French personalism. To distil from this diversity of approaches a coherent picture of personalism – which draws together its strands and is consistent with the conceptualization I have provided of personhood – a simple distinction can be made between strict personalism and broad personalism.[32] These forms draw respectively on, and complement, relational and existential constructions of personhood (Chapter 6). Both forms explicate respect for the centrality and absolute value of the person. My integrated focus here, of course, is on personalism in health care. This personalism centres on the relationship of the human persons of the clinician and patient to each other as human beings who, as emphasized by philosophers such as Martin Buber and Emmanuel Levinas, cannot be fully human on their own. Only through their interaction can the clinician and patient continue to experience and grow who they are in order to become and self-realize their shared nature as persons. What is real for them is (inter)personal as they interpret the world in terms of related personalities and possibilities.

In these terms, person-centred health care seeks to understand and manage issues that, although largely hidden from view, are basic to all persons. These issues relate to the meaning, value and dignity of personhood. Hence, in depathologizing, normalizing and destigmatizing illness, person-centred health care moves from labelling conditions, like insomnia, as things that define people to concretely describing persons as having difficulty sleeping. It sheds light on how they expect their health and health care to be, so that the content of this care, even when it is standardized, feels personalized. Such care respects what it means to each person to action their capabilities, move beyond current difficulties and flourish as whole persons; that is, in everyday behaviour, to organize their life around goods that enable them to be(come) the best persons they can in a life they live well.

To these ends, person-centred health care highlights the uniqueness and originality, but also the incompleteness and potentiality, of each person – who *sui generis* has a personal identity, including a history – in moral, social and spiritual life. The shared experience of personhood binds all these persons together in celebration of their wholeness and nobility as bearers of ethical–moral values in everyday life. From these values and for persons to live them, person-centred health care expects these persons to develop and manifest their capabilities for moral character. These acts, in the situation at hand, motivate and enable persons to take the time to stop, think about and appreciate what it means to them to live well; to know, actualize and be true to who they are and want to become; and to feel a personal sense of wholeness, harmony and unity in facing their goals and challenges.

Personalism thus distinguishes person-centred health care from patient-centred health care in two main ways. First, emphasizing the ubiquity of the person, rather than patient-centricity, person-centred health care socially valorizes the person as being above divisions of role, function and social and health status. At the same time, person-centred health care can move between social roles like patienthood and clinicianship. I see these roles in the manner of the ancient Roman philosopher and political theorist, Cicero. For Cicero, the social role was a mask that is not, in itself, inauthentic – a concealment of a true self. Rather, *the mask forms a proper part of the person*. The role, of which the mask is constitutive, is a 'person-al' category of value and meaning, which represents 'an aspect of being [of the person] rather than an exposition or dissimulation of that person'.[33] This aspect sanctions the clinical intimacy of the patient–clinician relationship. Incomplete however, the role cannot do justice to the full nature and authentic development of the person. So, the principal focus of health care production shifts from social roles to persons *in toto*. In these terms, person-centred health care underscores persons as whole beings who perform social roles, among other things; share the same basic human condition; are fundamentally equal and are becoming alike through convergence of their socially determined identities.[34] They have rights and duties principally as persons who happen to occupy particular roles. This perspective indicates a need to scrutinize the assumptions underlying those roles and indeed to think beyond the roles.

In patient-centred health care, by contrast, the roles themselves are primary, totalizing and hegemonic relative to other expressions of social life. The role reduces the person situationally to an embodied social function of an individual: a patient or clinician. The role-part of each individual is absolutized at the expense of the whole person within social and service contracts. Put simply, therefore, the role defines the person. *The person is their role*, and only implicitly and secondarily, are roles and functions recognized convergently to describe persons.[35] Roles subordinate personhood to the social order by reducing personhood to its aspect – the role persona that, presented to the world, defines each person's social identity. This state resembles pre-Christian antiquity when the persona of actors carried the double meaning of the social role and the person playing it. The roles themselves, moreover, are structured and ordered, with patient-centred health care openly privileging the welfare of the patient to which the clinician is a means.[36] I have attempted to show that for advocates of person-centred health care, by contrast, the meanings of the concepts of role and person are not the same – since the role is merely part of the person – and nor is the fundamental welfare of patients greater than that of clinician. Both sets of participants are valued ends in themselves. From this perspective, over-attention to the social mask of the role distracts attention from, and weakens respect for, the ability of persons to develop fully and express their unique inner selves, which contributes to the impersonalism evident in modern health care. Person-centred health care restricts this development, for example to interpreting and negotiating expectations of the social role.

Second, personalism re-visions role boundaries between patients and clinicians, in terms of the inclusive moral space or territory of personhood in health care. This space does not reduce personhood to 'a transaesthetic realm of indifference'[37] to the role differences between patients and clinicians. Rather, despite the interdependence of these persons whose roles distinguish them as different, role convergence is re-scoping these roles and exposing a common humanity expressive of moral equality. In clinical encounters this humanity focuses less on the illness narrative of the patient than their life narrative. The latter narrative reveals the larger history, personhood and human needs of the patient in relation to the clinician. Self-constructed in storied accounts, the clinician and patient therefore create space for communion and relational knowing, which go beyond instrumental benefits such as improving a nosological diagnosis and enable both parties to flourish.

They can flourish because their social engagement through shared personhood emphasizes the mutuality and reciprocity of their relationship as a clinician and patient who, being persons, have intrinsic dignity, experience themselves as social beings and yet continue to become more than their roles. In an organic, 'double relation',[38] the patient and clinician relate as persons both to each other in nature (as well as, in some versions of personalism, with a divine person beyond nature) and to health care as a whole. Personalism therefore underpins health care as a unified state of contingent relations, elegantly captured in two African expressions: '*batho pele*', meaning 'people first', and '*unmuntu ngumuntu ngabantu*', meaning, 'I am because we are'.[39]

Moral equality

'Virtue', recognized Mary Wollstonecraft, 'can only flourish among equals.' Person-centred health care has an ethos that values highly the attribution of equal respect and concern for the welfare of all persons. On the basis of justice, including fairness and inclusiveness, this egalitarian position assumes that all persons existentially share the same basic moral status. However, was Josef Mengele – the 'Angel of Death' – Hippocrates' moral equal? Answering 'yes' sounds implausible but pertains only to both men having existed as human persons. In respect of this personhood they were at least potential moral agents with inherent and hence invariable moral worth. This worth minimally justified equal *consideration* of their moral interests. Here I am suggesting that their competing equal interests deserved equally fair hearings in moral and other courts of consideration. However, whilst entitled to participate there on an equal moral basis, they might or might not each be found there to have fulfilled capabilities for full personhood. Eluding capture and legal trial, Mengele was judged at least in the social court of universal morality, if not his inner court of conscience, to have perpetrated heinous, immoral acts that disentitled him to socially sanctioned rights with which all persons equally begin their lives.

Beyond role convergence, patients and clinicians therefore exist as persons – vulnerable to disease and death. They warrant equal opportunity as moral equals to maximize their capabilities to partner freely and reciprocally in health care. Contrary to the physician, Thomas Percival – the author of perhaps the first modern code of medical ethics – moral equality does not result from the clinician 'descending' to the level of the patient. Other things being equal, the clinician and patient are *already* moral equals. Thus, the welfare of clinicians, like that of other professionals such as teachers and police officers, is not necessarily less important than that of those they serve. Clinicians may experience less misfortune than patients but the point of equality and the justice it fosters is not to compensate for bad luck but rather to recognize that all persons are free to have their moral interests count. As an inclusive quality of identity, the concept of personhood challenges the assumption – common until the recognition, in the eighteenth century, of natural rights – that 'human beings are unequal by nature'. All persons remain ultimately free to give meaning to their life despite differences between them.

Compared with patient-centred health care, this model brings the clinician out of the shadow of the principle of primacy of patient welfare to join the patient in the light of personhood cast by the principle of moral equality. Putting first the welfare and interests of patients uses inequality to promote equality, as noted earlier, which violates the commitment to social justice in health care provision. It also harms clinicians because it subordinates their interests and is morally blind to their suffering and its implications for patients. It can directly harm patients because paternalistically privileging patients can patronize them; put unrealistic expectations on them; and weaken their ability to look outside themselves and empathize with, and express care to, clinicians.[40]

I noted above that, as a value of person-centred health care, equality underpins the virtue of justice. Objectively good, justice is important independently of its relation to the (subjective) moral interests of persons. However, justice supports the principle of moral equality. Assuming that 'all who count, count equally', this principle gives equal moral weight to optimizing the moral interests of all persons, and at minimum ensures no party is worse off in this respect. Removing any tendency of clinicians to act against the best interests of vulnerable patients, its focus on equality of *moral* interests avoids irrational, antisocial and immoral interests. As subjectively rational preferences, moral interests are 'prudentially comparable' or 'relevantly similar' in having similar moral value and a universal aspect. For example, all persons share equal interests minimally in not suffering and maximally in flourishing in their situation. To such ends, I will illustrate equality in mutual trust and reciprocated caring.

Mutual trust

Patient-centred health care emphasizes respect for patient autonomy as a bulwark against deception and coercion; as a precondition for patients trusting themselves and others, including the clinician; and to enable patients to realize their capabilities. However, constructing patient autonomy as agency can conflict with patient welfare. One reason is that, potentially opposing the motives and preferences of the clinician, this construction can stretch patients' capabilities and invite abdication of clinician responsibilities. Patients can be empowered to increase decision-making control where they can have expertise, but in other areas the clinician's expertise needs to prevail. In practice therefore, clinicians tend to restrict patient autonomy largely to accepting or refusing the care that, as clinicians, they are willing to offer. This care includes resources such as tests, prescription medications and information. Clinicians select what information to give and how to maximize patients' welfare, where 'full disclosure of information [to patients] is neither definable nor achievable; and even if it could be provided, there is little chance of its comprehensive assimilation'.[41] When non-treatment would harm others, provisos that excuse clinicians from obtaining consent make consent 'generally rather than invariably necessary'.[41] Thus, despite respect for patient autonomy, autonomy is vested more in clinicians than patients.

In this context, although most patients trust clinicians to act in their best interests, concern is growing that this trust has been declining over recent decades,[42] especially at an institutional and systems level.[43] When clinicians become indiscernible from the system in which they work, modern patients may perceive them to be untrustworthy, for example in providing services of uncertain clinical benefit and in implementing policy demands to deliver whole population health care that may benefit the community more than most patients.[44] It is not that patients dispute the public interest. Rather, what patients need to trust is that clinicians will act prudently, openly and with compassion to provide the most accessible and effective personal care, and at least individualize the delivery of population health care. In not resisting structural and systemic pressures to share their control over the terms, conditions and content of their work, clinicians can look untrustworthy. They can look unreliable in their commitment to personal care amid forces, like fragmentation of care, that increasingly turn them into moral strangers. For such reasons, public trust in the health professions appears fragile, potentially reducing the placebo effect, patient disclosure and adherence to health care treatment,[45] and weakening the trustworthiness of patients themselves to contribute to a trusting patient–clinician relationship.

Person-centred health care recognizes that the current minimal conception of patient autonomy is insufficient to meet the need of clinicians and patients to depend on each other in relations of trust. Onora O'Neill[41] therefore argued for developing a right to principled autonomy that, grounded in principles of human obligation and guided by practical reason, fosters trustworthiness.

However, from the perspective of person-centred health care, any such right is irrelevant. It says nothing about whether the patient or clinician who acts autonomously and in a trustworthy manner in particular circumstances has trustworthiness as a motivation – and can be trusted therefore to continue to appear trustworthy-like. Similar to the model of beneficence-in-trust, person-centred health care emphasizes: trust in persons out of concern and respect for their autonomy in terms of agency and authenticity; welfare interests; and other foundational values such as steadfastness. Such values underpin the development of virtues including good faith and fidelity, within social relations and structures that facilitate taking right actions for the right reasons. Increasing the trustworthiness of clinicians will help patients to trust them[46,47] amid the general failure of health care interventions to increase patient trust in clinicians.[48] Strengthening this trust may also enhance clinicians' self-trust, self-esteem and motivation to trust patients, boosting trust by patients in clinicians and themselves through a virtuous cycle. Exemplified by appropriate decision-making modes like shared decision-making, such mutual trust could improve cooperation, reduce the need for monitoring[49] and construct normativity in terms of the interconnectedness of the clinician and patient.

Reciprocated caring

As foundational or ethically basic human values, care and caring lie at the relational heart of both person-centred health care and patient-centred health care as moral enterprises. However, patient-centred health care emphasizes the care of the patient – whether through clinician care of the patient or through patient self-care. As such, patient-centred health care first fails to acknowledge the complex and multifaceted nature of care as an interdependent moral relation between persons within clinical encounters. Furthermore, it views care provision as a professional activity and caring as a gift. In contrast, person-centred health care views caring as an authentic mode of existence by whole persons who recognize each other as moral equals and participate in dialogical relation to each other – in what Martin Buber described as the 'I–Thou' relation – whose centre lies in the space between them. For mutual security, caring in this relation is personal and reciprocal, which widens the one-sided focus of patient-centred health care. Affirming the importance of giving as well as receiving care can take place from clinician to patient, patient to self, clinician to self and patient to clinician. By respecting the interdependence of care for, and by, patients and clinicians – and by dignifying the freedom of both parties to choose to participate or not in caring behaviour – reciprocated caring makes these persons important.

Reciprocated caring also avoids the objection that an ethics of care neglects justice, since reciprocated care unites the virtues of justice and humanity. Beyond these virtues, mutuality of care further indicates and maximizes the reach of other virtues to which clinicians and patients can aspire. These virtues include: kindness and compassion – as constructed in the form of empathy for others through participation in their difficulties; the courage to give and receive care, despite the knowledge that care can produce the opposite effect to that intended; gratitude as a reason for the norm of reciprocity or mutual benevolence; and perhaps even friendship. The notion that the physician and patient can be friends has attracted support but also criticism, for example from Kathryn Montgomery who prefers a medicine of neighbours. However, the clinician and patient are often more intimate than neighbours, though their relationship as moral equals is one in which they can care about and, within their capabilities, take care of each other and themselves through giving as well as receiving care. It follows that reciprocated caring and the virtues it tends to promote, and be reproduced by, draw on an ethic of care that resembles and may be subsumed under the more comprehensive theory of an ethic of virtue.

Seldom drawing on care literature from political and feminist theory and philosophy, patient-centred health care lacks person-centred health care's clear connection with care ethics or virtue ethics. Indeed, care ethics was developed because other ethical theories, which better describe patient-centred health care – for example in emphasizing the duty of persons to follow rules – tend to neglect the importance of care in moral life. They have taken for granted the fact that persons 'are not abstract individuals who morally relate to each other [by] following principles such as justice and nonviolation of autonomy'.[50] This implicit consideration of care, and its regulative potential to support the flourishing of persons by balancing their emotions and reasoning, may help to explain why patient-centred health care has been an ineffective bulwark against forces pulling in other directions. These forces include the depersonalizing high tide of evidence-based medicine and the perspective that caring is commonly a vice, naively condoning favouritism and injustice, which may promote a slave morality – an attack motivated by resentment toward the 'medical–scientific model' among groups such as nurses. [51]

Pæanism

Echoing Francis Peabody's[52,53] end-of-life expositions on caring for the patient, proponents of person-centred health care ask, 'Where lies the soul of the clinic?' The spiritual desert that health care is becoming drains the vital spirit of persons whereas, explained the Islamic scholar, Rumi, 'When you do things from your soul, you feel a river moving in you, a joy.' Health care can enable clinicians and patients to rediscover the joy that celebrates being alive and with others. Whilst experiencing life as meaningful, clinicians and patients need this joy – including attributes of vitality such as engagement, sense of purpose, humour, self-esteem and resilience.

With such joy they can flourish by setting and realizing situationally meaningful goals, even and perhaps especially in the face of adversity and disability. As an integrated system of total care, person-centred health care welcomes this challenge of rediscovering the soul of health care. Besides involving care 'of the person, for the person, by the person, and with the person', it moves care *beyond* the person in their circumstances. It reclaims health care's spiritual roots in ethical values that underpin virtues like gratitude, courage and humour.[50] Such virtues lose force without the energy of joy from within, which empowers the person to live optimally.

This interrelationship of virtue and joy makes person-centred health care a pæan to an ethics that praises and celebrates human life and the virtues. Person-centred health care delights, for example, in personal caring – through the art of joyful caring and self-transcendence. No such acclamation of life characterizes patient-centred health care, which lacks an explicit emphasis on virtue and the vitality of morality even, and perhaps especially, in the midst of human pain and suffering. Instead, it mundanely and ambiguously focuses on putting first the welfare of patients. Definitions of patient-centred health care further understate the joy of recognizing and responding to basic spiritual needs of persons for hope, meaning, purpose and connectedness in their lives.

I want to say more here about the virtue of joyful caring because it speaks most directly to how person-centred health care enlightens human life as a profound gift whose virtuous use can transcend distress and suffering. Person-centred health care enables clinicians as well as patients to cultivate and exemplify the attitude and practice of joyful caring for, and about, life and persons. For health workers, the National Patient Safety Foundation's Lucian Leape Institute has defined joy as 'the emotion of pleasure, feeling of success, and satisfaction [resulting from] meaningful work in health care'.[54] The Institute supports a patient-centred health system but does not explicitly relate joy in health workers to this system; yet recognizing their need, no less than that of patients, to find meaning in experiencing joy appears tacitly to advocate for person-centred health care.

Reasons for joyful caring include the belief that in joy is also courage and nobility,[55] which may directly and indirectly benefit patients in areas like pain, cardiovascular function and immunity.[56] At minimum, joyful caring – including humour, which, unlike irony, is never cruel – can defuse suffering and anger as totalizing experiences and enhance quality of life; since, even when we 'are at sea, and our ship is going down: better to laugh about it than cry'.[55] Even, and indeed especially at the end of life, good palliative care aims to respect personhood by assessing and maximizing daily sources of pleasure for the patient, such as massage.[57]

For the philosopher and Jesuit priest, Pierre Teilhard de Chardin, nobility comes from joy being 'the infallible sign of the presence of God'. Independent of religious faith, however, 'because there is always a hidden pain in humour, there is also sympathy'.[58] And the joyfully compassionate person benefits too. In humour they avoid taking themselves too seriously; relieve themselves from unreasonable self-expectation; and forgive themselves in social realms that can expect perfectionism.[59] Thus, integral to wisdom, humour can help to liberate patients and clinicians from, or at least reduce, their sorrow by making bearable what might otherwise seem unbearable, and equalize and enliven them as persons. As shown by the physician–social activist, Patch Adams, with humour the pain of clinical practice 'mostly doesn't sit as pain because that takes your energy: It is stimulus. Feel the pain; it's horrible. Don't hold the pain. Though it is painful, let's get to work. Let's get to work joyfully'.[60]

Other forms of joyful caring include the socio-psychological states of connectedness and flow. Persons can connect with activities, themselves and others. One form of connection with others is empathy. The virtuous clinician cares joyfully on the basis of natural or sincere empathy[61] rather than duty. Including 'congruence' between feeling and action,[62] empathic engagement can joyfully self-reward persons through energizing their focus on, and immersion in, fully absorbing, meaningful activities.[63] Examples of activities producing this flow can include listening with complete attention, and group singing that produces a self-transcendent state of fulfilment, even among persons with debilitating conditions like Parkinson's disease;[64] and Chapters 3 and 4 discussed transcendence as a psychospiritual practice for self-care by patients and clinicians respectively.[65]

Authenticity

The authentic self – the person that one really is when no one else is looking – may be a fundamentally pure and moral being or instead be an immoral brute; for a despot who acts in good faith is still a despot. However, whilst insufficient therefore as a virtue, authenticity is necessary for virtue. Virtue, without authenticity, ceases to be virtue. Accordingly, person-centred health care values authenticity highly, specifically as a dimension of autonomy. Authenticity enables clinicians and patients, in conscientious accordance with what they hold true, to choose to care and self-care in ways faithful to who they are and want morally to become. They authenticate themselves moreover by acting against the feigned virtue sometimes recommended to clinicians,[66,67] and to patients who, as Oscar Wilde warned, can be found 'pretending to be wicked and being good all the time'.

Patient centred health care emphasizes agency rather than authenticity as dimensions of autonomy. Yet, inauthenticity is pervasive in social life and has implications for health care practice. Inauthenticity includes deception through illusion and selective information exchange. Sceptics assert that arguments for authenticity are naive because inauthenticity lubricates the wheels of social intercourse. Inauthenticity can facilitate communication about difficult topics; limit harm to others and self; and be consensual, among persons who need and expect it for self-maintenance. Entangled with self-deception, it can be unavoidable. However, deception interferes with understanding the world and its dishonesty can be morally suspect. For example, consider lying, as a statement intended to mislead another person regarding what the liar believes is true.

Patient-centred health care does not endorse lying, of course, or condone clinicians withholding information that patients need to exercise autonomy – unless the clinician believes that the patient does not want to learn the truth; would be harmed by doing so; or would recognize the lie as a lie but believe it anyway in order to palliate the strain of accepting the truth. However, these exceptions reveal how patient-centred health care tolerates some deception by clinicians on the basis of a professional duty of patient care. This duty trumps deep values and conscientious objection by these clinicians. It reduces their authenticity to role obligations that restrict their behaviour and weaken their freedom to recognize and be true to themselves as individual human persons. In denying inner aspects of themselves, these clinicians allow inauthenticity or bad faith to emerge.

Person-centred health care, by contrast, recognizes that role authenticity is merely part of the authentic self of this person. It contends not that patient-centred health care disallows authenticity but rather that this care model values authenticity less, and in a less balanced manner, than does person-centred health care – a model that sets a higher, more just bar for deception to jump. Person-centred health care does not expect clinicians to lie for the sake of patients or deceive them from good intentions, even by faking empathy. It respects the right to stay silent but, in the absence of natural caring, it rejects surface acting from duty.[68] Instead, person-centred health care emphasizes a virtue ethic that, on the basis of moral equality, values double loyalty to moral interests of the patient and clinician. They are expected to be true to what they believe and – beyond this good faith – to have made transparent and mutually consented to any potentially harmful deception. Aesop's fable, *The Scorpion and the Frog*, suggests that it can be in the nature of people to deceive, but person-centred health care rejects this premise. To facilitate free choice, it fosters conditions and strategies for safe, honest, compassionate communication. To replace reflection of feeling that may be empathetic or not, such strategies include listening that is inherently empathetic to check perceptions of felt experience within an egalitarian climate of mutual trust.

In an age of growing mistrust by patients of health systems and of moral disengagement by clinicians, such strategies 'reframe the opposition between empathy and genuineness ... as a generative tension'.[69] They enable clinicians and patients to grow trust by developing 'authentic consciousness' of, and respect for, their own values and those of the other person.[70] Actions chosen, from silence to truth-telling, can then take place conscientiously and with sensitivity through moral practices like authentic caring and authentic compassion.[71] Evident here is fidelity, with temperance, to shared interests such as to minimize moral suffering from giving and learning the truth; and enabling the other to feel validated and empowered to share decision-making.

Therefore, regardless of Augustine's and Immanuel Kant's belief that persons are duty-bound to tell the truth – save no exceptions – good faith and truthful disclosure never sanction tactlessness, nor do they condone bad manners or carelessness that can be avoided. Person-centred clinicians aim to be as truthful as possible without compromising decency. Mindful that emotions can be revealed inadvertently, they openly speak to their emotions in ways that can be reasonably expected to heal patients, or at least not harm them, while helping themselves. Authenticity frees clinicians and patients to admit to each other their own frailty and vulnerability within clinical encounters. It frees them to admit to feeling disappointed or frustrated and indeed to cry as a healthy reaction to sadness. In contrast, while clinicians expect complete truthfulness from patients, patient-centred health care can require clinicians to disguise their own anguish, paternalistically to protect patients.

Consilience

Though sometimes cast as a science,[72] patient-centred health care has been quiet until recently on the importance of science in health care despite the shadow that science can cast over providing a caring service to the patient. Evidence-based medicine has endured the opposite problem. It has struggled to explain how to integrate research evidence situationally with other influences operating on medical decision-making, such as patients' values and preferences. As a constructive alternative to conflict, bridge-building has been suggested to depend on dialogue as a collaborative rather than oppositional form of public, social interaction to exchange perspectives, facilitate understanding and lessen mistrust. However, dialogue has not been apparent between proponents of evidence-based medicine and patient-centred health care, who have weakly held one another's beliefs to account. Scholars operating largely without affiliation to either model have therefore taken on the roles of critic and conscience for the good of society. These commentators (including me) have in particular used annual thematic issues of the *Journal of Evaluation in Clinical Practice* to debate evidence-based medicine.

Evidence-based medicine has reformulated itself in response but has become a misnomer since it no longer requires physicians to *base* medicine on evidence and still retains limited ability to construct medicine as a caring practice. Progress in modern health care has continued therefore to depend on marrying advances in science with equivalent respect for humanistic values like caring and the virtues for the sake of the patient and clinician. Integration has been suggested through models such as evidence-based patient choice[73] and evidence-based individualized care.[74] However, keeping the misleading 'evidence-based' prefix, these models are no more appropriate than the temporally limited, chronic care model.[75] In contrast, as argued above, person-centred health care synthesizes the sciences, represented by evidence-based health care; incorporates the ethos of care exemplified by patient-centred health care;[7,76] and adds the development of virtue that clinicians and patients need to live well for good reasons. Remedying the 'anti-professional agenda' that has tended to characterize evidence-based medicine and patient-centred health care,[76] person-centred health care humanizes personal health care, including precision medicine, by attending to beliefs, values and virtues of the clinician and patient.

What makes this synthesis possible is consilience, a model rejuvenated by Edward Wilson[77] and supported for use in health care practice.[78] A consilient model embraces integration and unity. It values and signifies a patchwork of explanation produced by weaving together potentially wide sets of knowledge like scientific empiricism and transcendentalism. Without necessarily agreeing with each other, these different sets meet or coincide where they can help to account for common outcomes such as welfare. I associate person-centred health care with a form of consilience that links independent yet also related perspectives into a web of strong personal beliefs.[79] In clinician–patient encounters, the intersection of these personal and subjectively rational beliefs may indicate a shared ability of persons, despite their potentially different world views, to function together within a common moral project in order to identify and address their common goals.

The beliefs may also converge with respect to perceived outcomes of shared interest and benefit. Pragmatic rewards of working together, therefore, may motivate persons to strive for joint excellence through bridging elucidated personal interests across borders, including science and humanism; science, faith-based traditions and virtue; and personal care and population care. As a consequence, consilience gives scope to rehumanize health care as a science-using practice, art, philosophy and moral enterprise. Responsive to diverse warrants for effective and ethical action, it offers scope to integrate knowledge fragmented by scholarship from potentially conflicting perspectives; frees health care to respect beliefs that cohere to satisfy moral interests, regardless of whether these beliefs are true or real; and avoids the polarizing premise that science constitutes a superior form of knowledge and privileged method for testing consilience. Virtues such as resourcefulness and tolerance of difference and uncertainty facilitate this synthesis, as evident in the biopsychosocial–spiritual model of care.[80]

Much discussion about this model relates to end-of-life issues. However, in contrast to its author I wish to recommend its relevance to all patients, not only those who are sick or at the end of their lives, as well as to others including clinicians. The model assumes that all persons are intrinsically spiritual, and spirituality is health care. Persons are spiritual because they are capable of first-person transcendental experience – independent of second-order religious revelation – and of having faith that this world makes sense, regardless of how it appears. They seek healing through health care to maintain and restore right relationships inside and outside the body and understand not only what medical afflictions take place and how, but also why. To be whole persons they can choose how science and spirituality can help to meet their existential and relational needs in different spheres of action. Insights of science and spirituality thus interpercolate as porous rather than impermeable social discourses that support interests of the whole person of the patient and clinician.

Compared with patient-centred health care, my version of consilience makes explicit how beliefs drawn from domains including science, spirituality and religion can come together to inform the development and practice of person-centred health care. It would be naive however, at least in the short term, to believe that patient-centred health care and evidence-based medicine will disappear. They can be expected to continue to grow their distinctive identities in order to survive external pressure for change and resolve implicit, value-based and epistemological differences between their conceptualizations of health care – which cannot be easily adjudicated. Preferring to speak largely in parallel monologues, they will continue to choose to lose potential benefits of recognizing and engaging publicly in a conversational pluralogue with person-centred health care.

Conclusion

This chapter has recommended a framework for conceptualizing person-centred health care. Suggested sets of core abstract values of person-centred health care were identified and examined for their ability to help define this framework and distinguish it clearly from patient-centred health care. At the same time, I have linked values of person-centred health care to the development of virtues characteristic of person-centred clinicians and their patients, whose commitment to welfare finds expression in becoming relationally the best persons they can in their everyday life. This personal flourishing for self-actualization emphasizes their recourse to the virtues, led by prudence, ahead of duty. Key virtues include justice and caring – in order to respect through joyful, reciprocated caring the value of the moral equality of all persons – in good faith and interdependently. I hope this discussion of person-centred health care as a virtue ethic grounded in a values-based framework will stimulate and guide serious debate, in particular about what person-centred health care is and what it asks of its practitioners, including patients. At the same time it provides a platform for considering what conditions are needed to implement and test its ability to satisfy its raison d'être. Such is the purpose of the next chapter.

References

1 Little M. Values, foundations and being human. In: Loughlin M, editor. *Debates in Values-Based Practice*. Cambridge: Cambridge University Press 2014; pp. 171–83.

2 Little M. Humanistic medicine or values-based medicine … what's in a name? *Medical Journal of Australia* 2002; 177: 319–21.

3 Little M, Lipworth W, Gordon J, Markham P, Kerridge I. Values-based medicine and modest foundationalism. *Journal of Evaluation in Clinical Practice*. 2012; 18: 1020–6.

4 Fulford KWM. *Moral Theory and Medical Practice*. Cambridge: Cambridge University Press; 1989.

5 American College of Physicians. Core values. 2015; Available at: www.acponline.org/about_acp/who_we_are/core_values/. Accessed 16 March 2015.

6 Little M, Lipworth W, Gordon J, Markham P. Another argument for values-based medicine. *International Journal of Person Centered Medicine* 2011; 1: 649–56.

7 Miles A, Mezzich J. The care of the patient and the soul of the clinic: person-centered medicine as an emergent model of modern clinical practice. *International Journal of Person Centered Medicine* 2011; 1: 207–22.

8 Rider E, Kurtz S, Slade D, Longmaid HE, Ho MJ, Pun JKH, Eggins S, Branch WT. The International Charter for Human Values in Healthcare: an interprofessional global collaboration to enhance values and communication in healthcare. *Patient Education and Counseling* 2014; 96: 273–80.

9 Eagleton T. The nature of evil. In: Zaleski P, editor. *The Best of Spiritual Writing, 2013.* London: Penguin 2012; pp. 10–20.

10 Beauchamp TL, Childress JF. *Principles of Biomedical Ethics.* Fifth edition. Oxford: Oxford University Press; 2001.

11 Damon W, Colby A. *The Power of Ideals.* Oxford: Oxford University Press; 2015.

12 Price T, Harrison T. What is character?: Virtue Ethics in Education. 2015; Available at: www.coursetalk.com/providers/futurelearn/courses/what-is-character-virtue-ethics. Accessed 16 March 2015.

13 Toon P. Towards a philosophy of general practice: a study of the virtuous practitioner. Occasional Paper 78. London: Royal College of General Practitioners; 1999.

14 Marcum J. *The Virtuous Physician.* Dordrecht: Springer; 2012.

15 Arthur J, Kristjánsson K, Thomas H, Kotzee B, Ignatowicz A, Qiu T. Virtuous medical practice. Birmingham: Jubilee Centre for Character and Virtues, University of Birmingham; 2015.

16 Campbell A, Swift T. What does it mean to be a virtuous patient? Virtue from the patient's perspective. *Scottish Journal of Healthcare Chaplaincy* 2002; 5: 29–35.

17 Walker R. Virtue ethics and medicine. In: Besser-Jones L, Slote M, editors. *The Routledge Companion to Virtue Ethics.* New York: Routledge 2015; pp. 515–28.

18 MacIntyre A. *After Virtue: A Study in Moral Theory.* Notre Dame, IN: University of Notre Dame Press; 1981.

19 Veatch R. Character formation in professional education: a word of caution. In: Kenny N, Shelton W, editors. *Lost Virtue (Advances in Bioethics, Volume 10).* Bingley: Emerald Group Publishing 2006; pp. 29–45.

20 Peterson C, Seligman M, editors. *Character Strengths and Virtues. A Handbook and Classification.* Oxford: Oxford University Press; 2004.

21 Lebacqzk K. The virtuous patient. In: Shelp E, editor. *Virtue and Medicine.* Dordrecht: Kluwer Academic Publishers 1985; pp. 275–88.

22 Howick J. *The Philosophy of Evidence-based Medicine.* Oxford: Wiley-Blackwell; 2011.

23 Djulbegovic B, Guyatt G. Epistemologic inquiries in evidence-based medicine. *Cancer Control* 2009; 16: 158–68.

24 Wyer P, Silva SA, Post S, Quinlan P. Relationship-centred care: antidote, guidepost or blind alley? The epistemology of 21st century health care. *Journal of Evaluation in Clinical Practice* 2014; 20: 881–9.

25 Epstein R, Street Jr. R. The values and value of patient-centered care. *Annals of Family Medicine* 2011; 9: 100–3.

26 Fox N. Postmodern reflections on 'risk', 'hazards' and 'life choices'. In: Lupton D, editor. *Risk and Sociocultural Theory: New Directions and Perspectives.* Cambridge: Cambridge University Press 1999; pp. 12–33.

27 Swanton C. Two problems for virtue ethics. In: Snow C, editor. *Cultivating Virtue: Perspectives from Philosophy, Theology, and Psychology.* Oxford: Oxford University Press 2014; pp. 111–34.

28 Callahan D. Universalism and particularism. Fighting to a draw. *Hastings Center Report* 2000; 30: 37–44.

29 Pellegrino ED. Medical ethics in an era of bioethics: resetting the medical profession's compass. *Theoretical Medicine and Bioethics* 2012; 33: 21–4.

30 Bauman Z. *Postmodern Ethics.* Oxford: Blackwell; 1996.

31 Kristjánsson K. Ten myths about character, virtue and virtue education – plus three well-founded misgivings. *British Journal of Educational Studies* 2013; 61: 269–87.

32 Williams TD. What is Thomistic personalism? *Alpha Omega* 2004; 7: 163–97.

33 Bartsch S. *The Mirror of the Self: Sexuality, Self-Knowledge, and the Gaze in the Early Roman Empire.* Chicago: University of Chicago; 2006.

34 Buetow S, Jutel A, Hoare K. Shrinking social space in the doctor–modern patient relationship: a review of forces for, and implications of, role convergence. *Patient Education and Counseling* 2009; 74: 97–103.

35 Mead N, Bower P. Patient-centredness: a conceptual framework and review of the empirical literature. *Social Science and Medicine* 2000; 51: 1087–110.

36 Tanenbaum S. What is patient-centered care? A typology of models and missions. *Health Care Analysis* 2015; 23: 272–87.

37 Baudrillard J. *The Transparency of Evil.* London: Verso; 2009.

38 Quadrio P. Hegel's relational organicism: the mediation of individualism and holism. *Critical Horizons* 2012; 317: 317–36.

39 van Stadie W. African approaches to an enriched ethics of person-centred health practice. *International Journal of Person Centered Medicine* 2011; 1: 14–17.

40 Fourie C. What is social equality? An analysis of status equality as a strongly egalitarian ideal. *Res Publica* 2012; 18: 107–26.

41 O'Neill O. *Autonomy and Trust in Bioethics.* Cambridge: Cambridge University Press; 2005.

42 Beard ELJ. Consumer trust in healthcare organizations is waning. How will 21st century leaders bridge the gap? *Nursing Administration Quarterly* 2004; 28: 99–104.

43 LaVeist T, Nickerson KJ, Bowie JV. Attitudes about racism, medical mistrust, and satisfaction with care among African American and white cardiac patients. *Medical Care Research and Review* 2000; 57: 146–61.

44 Rose G. *The Strategy of Preventive Medicine.* Oxford: Oxford University Press; 1992.

45 Lee Y, Lin J. Linking patients' trust in physicians to health outcomes. *British Journal of Hospital Medicine* 2008; 69: 42–6.

46 Kukla R. Conscientious autonomy: displacing decisions in healthcare. *Hastings Center Report* 2005; 35: 34–44.

47 Lee YY, Lin JL. Trust but verify: the interactive effects of trust and autonomy preferences on health outcomes. *Health Care Analysis* 2009; 17: 244–60.

48 Rolfe A, Cash-Gibson L, Car J, Sheikh A, McKinstry B. Interventions for improving patients' trust in doctors and groups of doctors. *Cochrane Database of Systematic Reviews* 2014, 3; doi:10.1002/14651858.CD004134.pub3.

49 Thom D, Wong S, Guzman D, Wu A, Penko A, Miaskowski C, Kushel M. Physician trust in the patient: Development and validation of a new measure. *Annals of Family Medicine* 2011; 9: 148–54.

50 Halwani R. Care ethics and virtue ethics. *Hypatia* 2003; 18: 161–92.

51 Paley J. Caring as a slave morality: Nietzschean themes in nursing ethics. *Journal of Advanced Nursing* 2002; 40: 25–35.

52 Peabody F. The care of the patient. *Journal of the American Medical Association* 1927; 88: 877.

53 Peabody F. The soul of the clinic. *Journal of the American Medical Association* 1928; 90: 1193–7.

54 Roundtable on Joy and Meaning in Work and Workforce Safety. Through the eyes of the workforce: creating joy, meaning and safer health care. Boston: Lucian Leape Institute and the National Patient Safety Foundation; 2013.

55 Comte-Sponville A. *A Short Treatise on the Great Virtues. The Uses of Philosophy in Everyday Life.* London: Random House; 2003.

56 McCreaddie M, Wiggins S. The purpose and function of humour in health, health care and nursing: a narrative review. *Journal of Advances in Nursing* 2007; 61: 584–95.

57 Nakano K, Sato K, Katayama H, Miyashita M. Living with pleasure in daily life at the end of life: recommended care strategy for cancer patients from the perspective of physicians and nurses. *Palliative and Supportive Care* 2013; 11: 405–13.

58 Hong HV, Hong EH, editors. *Kierkegaard's Writings, XII: Concluding Unscientific Postscript to Philosophical Fragments, Volume 1. Soren Kierkegaard.* Princeton, New Jersey: Princeton University Press; 1992.

59 Blustein J. Doctoring and self-forgiveness. In: Walker RL, Ivanhoe PJ, editors. *Working Virtue: Virtue Ethics and Contemporary Moral Problems.* Oxford: Clarendon Press 2007; pp. 87–112.

60 Adams P. Patch Adams – End of Capitalism – Revolution of Love. 2011; www. youtube.com/watch?v=Gm4l-vIaQ1I.

61 Noddings N. *Caring: A Feminine Approach to Ethics and Moral Education.* Berkeley: University of California Press; 1984.

62 Rogers C. *A Way of Being.* Boston: Houghton Mifflin; 1980.

63 Csíkszentmihályi M. *Creativity: Flow and the Psychology of Discovery and Invention.* New York: Harper Collins; 1996.

64 Buetow S, Talmage A, McCann C, Fogg L, Purdy S. Conceptualizing how group singing may enhance quality of life with Parkinson's disease. *Disability and Rehabilitation* 2014; 36: 430–3.

65 Davidson JE, Palmer B. Is responsiveness to family wishes an expression of professional transcendence? *Critical Care Medicine* 2009; 37: 760–1.

66 Radden J, Sadler J. Character virtues in psychiatric practice. *Harvard Review of Psychiatry* 2008; 16: 373–80.

67 Faust H. Kindness, not compassion, in healthcare. *Cambridge Quarterly of Healthcare Ethics* 2009; 18: 287–99.

68 Prose N, Brown H, Murphy G, Nieves A. The morbidity and mortality conference: a unique opportunity for teaching empathic communication. *Journal of Graduate Medical Education* 2010; 2: 505–7.

69 Arnold K. Behind the mirror: reflective listening and its tain in the Work of Carl Rogers. *Humanistic Psychologist* 2014; 42: 354–69.

70 McCormack B. A conceptual framework for person-centred practice with older people. *International Journal of Nursing Practice* 2003; 9: 202–9.

71 Scott J. Authentic compassion. *Obstetrics and Gynecology* 2013; 122: 148–50.

72 Epstein R. The science of patient-centered care. *Journal of Family Practice* 2000; 49: 805–7.

73 T. Hope. Evidence based patient choice. London: King's Fund; 1996.

74 Westrom K, Maiers M, Evans R, Bronfort G. Study protocol. Individualized chiropractic and integrative care for low back pain: the design of a randomized clinical trial using a mixed-methods approach. *Trials* 2010; 11.

75 Wagner E. Chronic disease management: what will it take to improve care for chronic illness? *Effective Clinical Practice* 1998; 1: 2–4.

76 Loughlin M. What person-centered medicine is and isn't: temptations for the 'soul' of PCM. *European Journal for Person-Centered Healthcare* 2014; 2: 16–21.

77 Wilson EO. *Consilience. The Unity of Knowledge.* New York: Alfred Knopf; 1998.

78 Djulbegovic B, Morris L, Lyman G. Evidentiary challenges to evidence-based medicine. *Journal of Evaluation in Clinical Practice* 2000; 6: 99–109.

79 Boudon R. Beyond rational choice theory. *Annual Review of Sociology* 2003; 29: 1–21.

80 Sulmasy D. A biopsychosocial-spiritual model for the care of patients at the end of life. *Gerontologist* 2002; 42: 24–33.

8 Implementing person-centred health care

Introduction

Over a century ago, Francis Peabody told the Boston Medical Society, 'We must not forget in treating diabetes that we are treating a man [*sic*] and not a disease.' Candy's patient-centred primary care physician understood this message in caring for Candy, a 63-year-old woman who had lived with Type 2 diabetes for six years. Candy had continued to visit him, commonly complaining of feeling tired and a little down. Lacking support from family and friends for self-care, she had been unable to stop smoking and follow her prescribed diet, exercise and oral agents for her poorly controlled diabetes. At her last visit, Candy had requested a care plan to help her feel better without stopping smoking and aiming for the strict blood sugar control that her physician favoured. He recognized that Candy, being still relatively healthy, occupied a 'grey zone' in which the appropriate intensity of glycaemic control to aim for was uncertain. He respected her autonomy by undertaking to explore with her the changes she was willing to make and how they might benefit her. He did not recognize that his remit was less to give Candy control over her condition than to help align their shared interests to optimize joint benefit.

Today a *person-centred* physician is covering for Candy's usual physician when she visits for care of the same problems associated with her living with diabetes. After listening to Candy's story, the locum suggests that they aim to achieve what she and her regular physician *both* want – an approach tailored to suit Candy, yet also comprising ways that each party endorses for its potential to help Candy feel better and assist her physician to satisfy his moral interests in their mutual care. The locum physician and Candy agree to try to create such an integrated 'win-win' plan for caring for her diabetes. Faithful to their joint interests it will focus on activities that Candy can enjoy and conduct on her own and with others to improve her life, reduce her need for health care from her usual physician and optimize his ability to help both of them. The locum asks Candy what activities are fun and not fun respectively for her. He learns that walking hurts her knees but she likes watching tennis. Candy finds cooking and exercise boring but enjoys 'surfing' the Web. They identify Candy's interest in digital media as a resource for her self-care. The locum encourages Candy to join an online social support network of people with similar experience of living with diabetes. She can connect anytime with this group to feel less isolated and, with compassion, assist others who are like her. The network may also help her to learn about active video games she can play, standing or seated, at home or outdoors using her smartphone. Playing such games will add a physical activity component to her lifestyle and provide unobtrusive feedback to help monitor her health. The locum also mentions online sites and management apps, for example offering fun meal ideas using her favourite foods to help manage her diabetes. All these plans for Candy's self-care will assist her usual physician, who will revisit her smoking after she has implemented healthy but pleasurable habits for eating and physical activity.

A second story further illustrates how person-centred health care can differ from patient-centred health care. Rudy is the type of patient that many physicians would describe as a 'problem patient'. He always seems to present for care in a state of crisis, make clinically inappropriate demands and then react with anger and other negative emotions to the inability of his physician to meet these demands. His physician recognizes Rudy's anger as pain and strives to understand and manage it with him. The pain they recognize is Rudy's pain and the care they produce is *for* Rudy. However, the physician feels lonely, emotionally exhausted and frustrated as Rudy's behaviour continues to challenge her. To break herself free – and help Rudy – she makes her care person-centred by being courageously true to who she is as a person and gaining Rudy's permission to tell him how their relationship makes her feel. She gently confesses to Rudy that it hurts her to feel some of his pain and to know that her feeling hurt weakens her care for him. Her emotional nakedness helps to establish with Rudy the credibility she needs in order to grow mutual trust between them and co-produce care for their shared benefit.

These stories illustrate how my conceptualization of person-centred health care could look in practice. For such care to come fully to light, there is a need to focus on and foster preconditions for implementing it. Cultural and structural arrangements are needed to organize social development and social life in ways that cultivate and facilitate virtues that clinicians and patients require for this care. Obstacles to meeting this need include the difficulties of enhancing deep values, character and intrinsic motivation within existing social structures, including families and the education and health sectors.

Regulatory and bureaucratic health systems, for example, retrofit concern for character and motivation into structures that limit clinical and patient freedom and moral action by standardizing social roles. For example, more than one fifth of experienced physicians in the United Kingdom have recently reported that workplace arrangements 'sometimes' or 'often' make it difficult for them to live up to their standards of good character.[1] Intended to protect the public, structures including clinical practice guidelines, pay-for-performance programmes, and documentation and public reporting requirements can sometimes perversely influence clinical practice. Such arrangements can incentivize measurement fixation and 'gaming'; increase administrative costs; restrict the time that clinicians, struggling to protect their professional authority, can spend with patients;[2] and limit patients' opportunities for moral action. Without losing the need for external accountability in health care, humanizing health care will require creating social structures and institutions that intrinsically motivate health care teams, including patients, to make moral decisions – for systems are only as good as the people using them.

Accordingly, it is necessary to empower people to share control over, and responsibility for, their choices, which can be more complex than rules and principles can codify. This need will require a cultural shift in society to redefine social roles and relationships and develop dimensions of personhood within social institutions associated with health care, families, education and technology. Such change is key to clinicians and patients developing good character as a public and private concern.

As relational beings, persons can best address this concern through participating in communities to create 'social and political arrangements that cultivate in citizens certain habits and dispositions, or civic virtues'.[3] Progress toward these virtues will enable persons to progress toward actualizing their moral capabilities and promoting civic life and the common good. Implemented across public–private spaces, person-centred health care ceases then to overwhelm, since it legitimates moral governing by people as a collective responsibility in the realm of citizenship. This perspective resonates with Paul Ricoeur's unwillingness to countenance people's withdrawal from political and social engagement. Collective engagement by persons requires their participating in partnerships for social change.

Such partnerships can connect service users and clinicians, for example through collaborative research approaches like Experience-based Co-design of services and care pathways. This approach involves staff, patients and even their carers in sharing their care experiences and working together to design, implement and reflect on public service improvements responsive to these experiences.[4] Values clarification and values development enhance these processes by enabling participants to restructure systems that attend to what people care most about; for values are inculcated in people, not directly in systems. Everything flows from the person who, as Christian Smith notes, is 'constitutionally social by nature'.[5] For the common good of rehumanizing social life, people can be enabled to develop, recognize and draw on deep moral values to grow as persons and promote civic freedom through, and within, change to social systems. To imbue people with moral values and form their identity and 'social character', systems and institutions need to help them to develop their individual character.

This chapter will discuss potential strategies for implementing this conceptualization. I will suggest ways to create a subculture-environment of social structures and processes for developing the character of clinicians and patients to advance social relations for person-centred health care. Specifically, I will discuss areas of social life that present opportunities to develop these conditions. I will begin with infants' early character development through child-rearing, including potential benefit from religious upbringing. Building on this foundation are discourses and partnerships that can take place between families, schools and religious institutions to educate children in moral values and develop virtues. In health care, character education can further take place at young adult ages and through lifelong learning by health professionals and patients. Complementing character education and social reform is the potential for technology to mediate change, for example through informational media and the scope for moral bioenhancement and related advances to optimize moral being. I will discuss these openings for change before looking at how to review progress toward, and the impact of, implementing person-centred health care, and balance the welfare of patients and clinicians when their deep values differ.

Early character development

The genesis of moral character development is complex but may be evident from the time of birth, if not before. Evolutionary theory indicates that human beings have evolved to need responsive parenting.[6] Attachment theory and ethics of care similarly relate moral development early in life to infants' affective experience of protective social interactions with caregivers.[7] Research in developmental psychology suggests that in the first year of infancy, receipt of love and care stimulate the uncensored development of an early pre-moral sensibility.[8] As a psychological foundation for moral growth, this intuitive moral sense of how to act establishes in infants as they learn emotional and conceptual skills. Constitutive of a nascent understanding that other people have feelings, needs and intentions that can account for their actions, these skills support infants' prosocial behaviour. The skills can form part of a moral value system before five years of age, by which time children can perceive caregiver expectations to try to meet in order to be 'good'. This system can most easily develop in a stable and nurturing environment as reasoning grows during middle childhood and adolescence.

Children need to be able to access these conditions for their early moral development. Modern society invites concern that, through overprotection and underprotection of children, social changes threaten this ability.[9] These changes include increases in female participation in paid and unpaid work and a shift toward complex and varied family structures, associated for example with single parenthood and blended family households. Characteristic of these developments is the emergence of less clearly demarcated social roles, which reframe everyday tasks of caregiving and maintaining a home. Put simply, changing work demands, fluid family structures, and caregiving responsibilities risk colliding – and marginalizing children. In combining their work and caregiving, women in particular need to be able to access policy-supported social structures to help them care for themselves and others, including nurturance of the character of their children from an early age. Social policies to advance these goals could include flexible work arrangements; expansion of non-parental childcare; father involvement in caregiving; and home–school partnerships for character education.

In terms of childhood schooling, most parents see character education as a central role,[10] a role that also pleases children.[11] Even if families do not want character formally taught in schools – for example because character education is believed to be outside the purview of schools, to manipulate moral choices, to be anti-educational and to risk mistaking good behaviour for good character – character is ineluctably infused there through the ethos of the school and how its members interact with each other every day. The values and character that children develop link in turn to their cognitive development. For such reasons, as shown by a recent study of 68 United Kingdom secondary schools, children benefit educationally from training teachers to model good character in a school culture committed to whole character development.[12] Involving 255 teachers and over 10,000 14–15 year-olds, the study found that, with the right approach, 'any kind of school can nurture good character'. To prioritize moral education in British schools, changes recommended by the report may yield concrete political action; for example, a 2012 report by the All-party Parliamentary Group on social morbidity concurs that 'character and resilience' are essential roles of schools in enabling students to learn the meaning of a good life.

Religious education through schools and religious groups can also connect with the religious background of the home to support character education from young ages. Religious upbringing and religious education can deepen moral character development. It is no coincidence that Catholic education is a leader of person-centred education in Europe and the United States. Its authority reflects the concern of the Catholic Church for profound aspects of human nature and personhood, including the quest for transcendentalism through the relationship of the person to a divine presence and judge. Jewish people, among others, have also been saliently civic-minded and philanthropic in performing good deeds from Jewish values acquired through approaches such as person-centred values clarification (which balances cognitive and affective components of personality development).

Character education

Beyond the cultivation of character and virtue in childhood lie opportunities to refine these qualities at young adult ages. I wish to focus on clinical education, especially in medicine, and patient education as fields of moral practice that can support relationship-building in health care, as well as lifelong moral learning and character development. These fields expose role modelling of person-centredness by professional and academic disciplines, which social learning theory suggests underpins how persons learn most human behaviour. The concept of the person has been central to models of nursing practice.[13-17] And, with strong traditions in care practice, the humanities such as social psychology have also led developments in person-centred care, especially in areas like dementia.[18] In medicine, person-centredness has been conspicuous in family practice, psychiatry and palliative medicine.

Despite erosion of trust in the family physician as the patient's moral fiduciary, family practice as an ideal has long been a natural role model for person-centred health care. As Ian McWhinney[19] explained, 'Family physicians are committed to the person rather than to a particular body of knowledge, group of diseases, or special techniques.' However, despite its specialty focus and detractors,[20] psychiatry – rather than family medicine – has led internationally the revitalization of person-centred medicine. Palliative medicine also stands out as understanding how, as persons and moral equals, patients and clinicians can care deeply for themselves and each other.[21] Palliative care facilitates reciprocal caring by epitomizing situational and compassionate insight from experience into the meaning to persons of their lived world – insight engaging the emotions and motivating moral learning and action.

Character education in medicine

Medical education has been slow to become patient-centred and even slower to become person-centred. Nevertheless, person-centredness is beginning to achieve recognition as part of a global resurgence of interest in advancing education in medical ethics and professionalism through moral and character education. In 2010, a global independent Commission on the Education of Health Professionals for the twenty-first century called for 'nothing less than a remoralization of health professionals' education'.[22] Its report envisaged socializing students into professionals as ethical and enlightened change agents.[23] This vision is consistent with developing virtue in medical students from their time of recruitment.

Medical schools vary in how they select and teach medical students. Increasingly, some schools in a growing number of countries are taking account of academic and non-academic selection criteria like personal skills; qualities that indicate aptitude for well-formed character traits such as empathy; and students' backgrounds, with a view to promoting equality of opportunity as a democratic ideal destabilizing social privilege in medical education. Medical schools may then build, even at young adult ages, on the moral development of the students they recruit, or at least not train them out of their natural moral impulse for sensibility. The following discussion explores this educational influence against a backdrop of concern that medical schools too often deform rather than reform students' professional development of personal qualities, values and intellectual and moral virtues.

Education and training for medicine typically begin by providing students with expert knowledge and facilitating their linear acquisition of cognitive and technical competencies to apply rules, principles and codes of clinical and professional conduct. Two problems have arisen here. First, students have been taught what to know rather than to learn how to think when making clinical decisions.[24] To address this problem, students are now learning to draw on moral principles and good examples in a critical and disciplined manner to solve open-ended problems and justify their decision-making. Yet students can remain unclear, for example, how to develop and balance critical thinking against external constraints such as professional standards; other forms of medical authoritarianism, including a quest for clinical certainty in the obscured face of ambiguity and uncertainty;[25] and morally laden financial incentives, such as the promotional gifts that some drug companies may offer even to medical students.[26] Thus, a second problem has been a failure to train students to deal with such pressures, which can act against a critical stance, through developing good character and emotional intelligence.

Medical education has neglected such problems by not 'grappling with deep issues of value and character formation',[27] and their relevance to students' motives, whose impact cannot be easily assessed. Reasons may include the range of approaches to defining and assessing professionalism as a construct under threat,[28] and the virtues inviting ill-founded, negative connotations. In the United States, however, a national survey found that most medical students support character education 'as part of medical training'.[29] Despite this support, character education tends to be an 'add-on' to the students' training in medicine rather than the substance of, and integral to, their training.

Exemplifying this problem are siloed learning activities introduced from the social sciences, humanities and arts to develop students' personal and professional skills. Such activities can reduce morality to a competency informed by task-enabling skills dichotomized from, and taking a back seat to, teaching about the biomedical and clinical sciences in medicine.[30] Informative rather than personally transformative, the cognitive activities are insufficient in themselves to provide the comprehensive experience needed by students to cultivate a 'soul-changing' way of living. Indeed, socialization processes, including discrimination and teaching students by intimidating and shaming them (processes known as pimping), can undermine character education. During clinical rotations, for example, hospital culture can erode developing moral qualities like affective empathy as students progress through their medical training into their clinical years.[31] As a consequence, students can learn to tolerate unprofessional behaviour, become cynical, conform and self-care through non-reflective professionalism – characteristics hindering their wellness and personal and professional development. Reversing this experience requires culture change. Moral learning necessitates a community of practice that agrees on moral values and then, as Jack Coulehan[27] explains, lives and breathes them.

Internationally, a number of medical schools have been developing such a community oriented to training in, and practising the values of, person-centred medicine. Students learn to manage ethical dilemmas; avoid demoralization in dehumanizing learning environments; and flourish relationally, for example through reflecting on and discussing everyday interactions with each other, clinicians and patients. Examples of these schools are found at Lima's Peruana Cayetano Heredia University and, within Europe, at Milan's Ambrosiana University, Brest's Bretagne Occidentale University, Plovdiv's Medical University, the University of Zagreb and Madrid's Francisco de Vitoria University. Opening in 2010, following implementation of the Bologna process to modernize higher education and training in Europe, the last of these medical schools, for example, emphasizes person-centredness from the first undergraduate years. Its curriculum highlights scientific, clinical, human and relational dimensions of medical care. Also evident are person-centred learning sites outside medicine, for example in health sciences at Buskerud and Vestfold University College in southern Norway; in nursing at Edinburgh's Queen Margaret University; and in the domains of Business and Economics, for which the Catholic University of America has created a character-based school. Although a focus on character development appears commonly fostered in educational institutions with a religious ethos, the concern to revitalize character education also forms part of a larger, post-religious movement.[32]

Some other institutional role models in medicine do not explicitly identify with person-centred health care or a virtue approach to medical education, but exemplify educational practice consistent with both. Noteworthy here are opportunities offered nationally by the American Medical Student Association, including its Medical Humanities Scholars Program, book discussion webinars and Writers' Institute. Regionally in the United States, the Indiana University School of Medicine continues to demonstrate leadership in building a moral community for undergraduate medical education. Rather than adopt typical culture change interventions, such as the implementation of an organizational values statement top-down,[33] the School produces – as a curricular issue – transformative, organizational change to the meaning and moral practice of medical professionalism. A commitment to moral, professional and humane values promotes the virtues, as basic educational aims, to frame rule-based evaluations of actions. Sweeping and impressive changes made since 1999 warrant my further discussion of them.

The School has produced a competency-based formal curriculum that aligns with an enhanced, informal curriculum. Aiming to produce personal skills, the competencies developed by the formal curriculum link learning experiences between the biomedical and clinical sciences to character-building and moral action.[32] However, the School understands that, without a proper informal curriculum, these developments would lack sufficient cohesion to produce virtuous physicians. Thus, as the social space in which unintended learning takes place continuously outside the formal curriculum, an informal or hidden curriculum has been developed to foster an everyday learning 'climate of humanism'[34] – a respectful climate for culturally safe, healthy and caring relationships to reinforce the moral values and teaching of the formal curriculum. The result is the seamless and transparent integration of the two curricula for medical education. Learning activities reinforce this moral learning environment.

From daily experience of the informal curriculum, students produce independent journals in the formal curriculum. The journals provide an opportunity for the students to develop personal knowing through reflecting on their experience of seminal events that express varying degrees of professionalism and ethics. Small group discussions enable the students to practise mentor-supervised and facilitated discernment of, and reflection on, salient ethical issues, for example from edited and anonymized versions of narratives shared by other students. Therefore, rather than be merely instructed in good character, students learn about it by participating in activities conducive to its development. Opportunities for creative and arts-informed self-expression add to this experience. They grow students' narrative competence – 'the ability to acknowledge, absorb, interpret, and act on the stories and plights of others'[35] – through raising self-awareness for self-knowledge, personal growth and knowledge of others.[36] Critical here has been fostering an environment in which students, and teachers, can speak freely and openly but politely[37] to develop virtues less through studying them than practising living them; for, as Aristotle said, 'Our examination is not to know what virtue is, but to become good.'

So far, I have focused on undergraduate medical education. After medical school, physicians working in today's complex health care environment continue to need and benefit from lifelong education including moral and character development. They depend for their personal and professional growth on working in health care organizations and systems that operate on and exemplify person-centred values, and enable them consistently to practise these values. Opportunities for such work include collaborating with patients, exposure to professional role models and participating in live and online courses and activities like group discussions. Groups include small groups, such as Balint groups, and larger groups comprising 35–200 participants, such as Schwartz rounds of interdisciplinary and interactive case- or theme-based discussions of psychosocial and emotional aspects of patient care.[38] Before I discuss patient education per se, I want to elaborate on opportunities for small group learning during and after medical school.

Specifically, Havruta-style learning – a Jewish mode of learning in pairs – has been applied for millennia to textual study of the Old Testament and Rabbinical commentaries, but in recent times also to learning in non-Jewish settings such as the Law classroom.[39] After or before teacher-led learning, Havruta entails discussions in pairs (or small groups) in which each person, who may vary in level of knowledge and experience, shares responsibility for their own learning and for learning by their partner. In this partnership, Havruta 'removes dependence on a teacher to provide a final or "correct" answer. Serving as a guide and participant in the quest for understanding, the teacher becomes another seeker of the "truth"'.[39] Accordingly, Havruta answers the concern of Plato – in his Socratic dialogue, *Meno* – that virtue cannot be taught because teachers of 'human excellence' cannot be found, or are not available in sufficient number for the traditional Master–apprentice model of education. Beyond the text whose meaning is interrogated, Havruta does not depend on the teacher's constant presence. Discussants learn moral virtue by engaging critically but democratically and safely in three core sets of behaviour: listening and articulating; wondering and focusing; and supporting and constructively challenging. Their supervised peer learning enables a kind of cognitive apprenticeship in which students can learn from experienced others, besides the teacher. Disavowing a hierarchy of intellectual and moral capacity, this learning environment puts into action the moral equality of each person, who learns from, and even becomes the master for, the other. There is, likewise, scope for educating patients to partner with clinicians to clarify, question, develop and act on deep values in co-producing care.

The physical and social environment can interact to support this vision. Architecture and design can help to engineer shared moral values within clinics and other community spaces.[40] Clean, comfortable and welcoming waiting rooms facilitate moral–therapeutic goals for patient well-being and learning. Further supporting these goals are explanatory tools such as posters; brochures that list common questions and prompts for patients to use during clinical visits; and character literature, including fiction. Such positive distractions for patients can shorten perceived waiting times and support virtues like patience and politeness. Consulting rooms, in turn, offer settings not only for clinical practice but also for shared moral learning. For example, corner-to-corner seating with chairs of the same height support a non-clinical feel and model social justice by minimizing power differences. This safe arrangement of physical space is conducive to clinicians and patients modelling good character; and using verbal strategies such as appropriate use of storytelling and technology, and coached care programmes. Similar ecological principles support group teaching led by clinicians or patients in patient participation groups, peer support and advocacy groups, and social activity groups. In turn, patients (and clinicians) can create environments conducive to them acting well rather than badly.

Moral discomfort

Virtue takes time to develop. Repeated affirmation of the good, suggested Aristotle, makes it a disposition of personal habit. Critical to the need for practice, added Aristotle, is 'The pleasure or pain that accompanies the acts.'[41] According to Aristotle, pain 'moves us to refrain from what is noble', and indeed I have referred above to minimizing patient distress. However, a stimulus to moral action can also be pain or discomfort that comes from experience of adversity. I am not, of course, advocating for moral discomfort but I am suggesting that, when such discomfort presents, it can be potentially constructed as a moral resource – a resource that can be important to use because, as Helen Keller observed, 'Character cannot be developed in ease and quiet. Only through experience of trial and suffering can the soul be strengthened, ambition inspired and success achieved.' Chapter 2 discussed these issues for patients but they apply also to clinicians in training and practice. Clinicians can develop virtues like humility within a 'pedagogy of discomfort'[42] that values personal experience, or at least being reflective and responsive witnesses to experience, rather than just learned spectators.[43,44]

For people to learn, for example, how to value moral equality and develop the virtue of justice, they can draw on experience of having suffered in some way, such as from personal experience of inequality. Such experience indicates moral sensitivity that can elicit strong emotions, especially those consistently and firmly validated in the social milieu. These emotions can motivate persons to feel, reason and act in ways that validate their feelings and intuitions.[45,46] The more powerfully that people experience inequality as intuitively incompatible with a good life – as something repulsive that educates and pricks their conscience and especially their sense of vulnerability – the less likely they are to turn away from inequality. If the felt threat of inequality is strong enough, they will be moved not only to value equality strongly but also to practise deliberately their learnt skills to achieve it. Reinforcement of this value over time can lead them to cultivate the virtue of justice – to become fair persons who resist inequality within the constraints of their capabilities. A catalyst for change here is a developed conscience that wills persons to do what they deeply sense is morally right. Conscience is not infallible but, from an obligation to form one's conscience correctly,[47] person-centred health care requires exceptional circumstances before compelling people to act against their conscience.[48]

At places like medical school, meaningful experience of discomfort is likely to require careful exposure to, and reflection on, activities ranging from acquaintance with human cadavers to supervised engagement with ethical issues in diverse clinical settings from an early stage in the training. Vicarious experience; natural sentiment, including empathy; and the ability to bridge different symbolic spaces may also be developed, for example through reflective engagement with truth-telling, fictional narratives from literature, film, poetry and other arts, as well as in real sites for social learning; for example, first year medical students at Madrid's private Universidad Francisco de Vitoria visit a former Nazi death camp to help sensitize their appreciation of core values like moral equality, human dignity and the sanctity of life. The visit also highlights the importance of community service, a theme that schools can reinforce, for example through experience of volunteer work in places like hospices. However, I want to reiterate the daily need to enculturate moral learning in ordinary social behaviour.

Social character

Personal character development facilitates and is strengthened by the contextual development of social character through the solidarity and power of social movements. Persons experiencing psychosocial strain can draw strength from their values and virtues by mobilizing these broad social alliances. An 'injustice frame' can develop in this context to challenge powerful institutions and act on available opportunities and resources to risk progressive social change to relieve the strain. Through the social reorganization of institutions to achieve more human ways of living, people can develop the freedom and will to resist strain. While this freedom is socially and historically situated, it is also personal.

This conceptualization is relevant to how person-centred health care is reshaping role-person identities and human relationships in health care. The movement is promoting social and moral change at all levels of society to strengthen its own solidarity as a sociopolitical force for rehumanizing modern health care. To achieve this vision, person-centred health care is drawing on its deep values and resources to advocate for, and bring about, social change. Recognizing the importance but also the insufficiency of political change, it is promoting in health care and society as a whole the bottom-up development of conditions that put people first in a more human and virtuous world. Crystallizing and coordinating recent advocacy for person-centred health care initiatives have been change agents.

These agents have led with passion and skill to motivate and recruit like-minded others who have a stake in – and can develop, adapt and implement with them – a shared vision for growing person-centred health care. Andrew Miles and Juan Mezzich stand out internationally as two such pioneers. From inside health care, they have been assembling global groups of professionals with the authority and resources to facilitate training, research and scholarship in person-centred health care, and promote and accomplish policy decision-making to re-personalize modern health care. To advance this mission, Miles and Mezzich have established formal structures and processes of good governance; forged alliances with leading health care professional and patient organizations; established academic journals – respectively the *International Journal of Person-Centered Medicine* and *European Journal for Person Centered Healthcare*; stimulated the production of other academic and clinical texts; established social media activities; and organized international conferences and training courses. The conferences underpin plans for international meetings and publications to develop person-centred practice for specific health conditions and topic areas. Noteworthy also have been institutional leaders for change. Beyond the educational institutions noted above are pockets of research excellence such as the Gothenburg Centre for Person-Centred Care. It has used strategic funding to conduct research, produce educational resources and implement joint care programmes, particularly for persons living with long-term conditions.[48] Further opportunities for leadership by change agents include promoting collaboration among the groups committed to person-centred health care; expanding this model into acute health care settings, like intensive care,[49,50] and regions south of the equator; and integrating health care, the social sciences and the humanities as well as person-centred clinical practice and people-centred public health. In turn, developing person-centred health care will require scholarly works, such as this one and effective modes of dissemination such as social media. Also useful may be natural experiments such as paying patients[51] and clinicians to participate in approved forms of moral learning and moral reinforcement and to exercise virtue until virtue becomes its own reward.[52] Yet, even evolutionary change can evoke classic psychological reactions. As Arthur Schopenhauer observed, before every truth is recognized, it is ridiculed and opposed before becoming ultimately self-evident.

Moral bioenhancement and other technologies

Character development and implementing person-centred health care can further benefit from advances in biological and psychological understanding.

Such advances underpin how new and emerging health technologies are developed, assessed and applied. Including medicines, devices, procedures and information and communication systems, the technologies respond to the needs of individual users for self-directed learning of content of personal relevance. Non-personalized technologies complement this development, as when Internet users adopt online personas to construct and express themselves and gain insight into these processes. Traditional media and social networking are informing people of such technologies, which can then acquire autonomy of their own; be simultaneously enabling and constraining; and support character development, for example through moral bioenhancement.

Future technologies, particularly in genetics and neurobiology, may over-come limitations of the fundamental human biology of persons. Biomedical moral enhancements are currently possible only to a small extent but pharma-ceuticals in use may be impacting on moral agency and society. Thus, it seems plausible that developments in science may one day enable humankind to enhance (biologically based) personal capabilities and dispositions for socially sanctioned moral behaviour such as empathy, a sense of justice and spiritual and religious experience conducive to virtues like altruism.[53] However, the overall aim here is 'not to make persons virtuous but to make them better equipped to learn how to be virtuous'.[54] Human enhancement technologies may be needed to achieve this aim because traditional methods of moral enhancement, such as education, have been insufficiently effective.

This transhumanist vision of morally advanced human beings invites open-minded interest for its potential to support and augment the ability of moral education, upbringing, socialization and institutional reforms to help persons thrive and live well. More specifically, the project of moral bioenhancement could protect core liberal values and remodel moral psychologies. It could also remedy defective human nature and moral and psychological shortcomings exposed by human history; reduce criminality; support personal growth, cultivate wisdom through cognitive and moral flourishing; strengthen human dignity and quality of life; and avert threats to human extinction from immoral behaviour and major dis-asters. Nevertheless, moral bioenhancement is a controversial concept.[55]

The distinction between treatment and enhancement of 'normal' capabilities can be unclear. Of particular concern is that interventions identified as major enhancements could produce inauthentic persons who, assuming an essential self, are not themselves. In these terms, bioenhancement might diminish rather than improve human personhood, the meaning of which is constantly evolving. Critical post-humanists respond that identity is emergent or they avoid meta-physical debates about the nature of personhood by treating 'the "essential" attributes of the human being as already imbricated with other life forms'.[56] The risk remains that bioenhancements could revive an execrable ideology of selective, sociobiological rebirthing.[57] However, they would not then be *moral* bioenhancements, and the moral superiority of 'post-persons' would equip them *not* to threaten ordinary persons. Moral bioenhancements of persons – for example through psychopharmaceuticals, genetic modifications, or external devices – could thus be used safely and judiciously to support the human mind and learning.

This project will still need to resist and minimize unintended and undesirable side effects of bioenhancements designed to champion progress. To avoid hubris, humankind must use technology wisely in striving for moral excellence while recognizing that moral perfection is unattainable. Before bioenhancements can approach their moral potential, it will be necessary to elucidate the complex nature and mechanisms of moral thought and moral behaviour, and appraise the scope and capacity of bioenhancements to limit vices and cultivate virtues. It will also be important: not to misapply bioenhancements whose unregulated moral effects could vary in different situations; to minimize risks to personal freedom, moral diversity and debate; and to rejuvenate, not extinguish, egalitarian social and political ideals that health inequalities threaten from unequal access to technology. With these caveats, improvements in moral character, motivation and skills across the ethics–technology boundary could help people to function as digital moral citizens; that is, use digital sites and other new technologies ethically to manage basic problems of daily living and advance the human condition.

Indeed, users themselves require the new technologies to facilitate ethical practice, for example by enhancing morally appropriate virtual realities with a high degree of realism. Users' ability to personalize these realities by customizing online experience adds to this realism. Perceptual and interactive features of telemedicine and other virtual reality systems will progressively resemble the real world for each person in an expanded range of settings. However, clinicians and patients will need to reconsider what it means to 'see' and be present with each other during virtual visits. If these visits aim to deepen empathic connection, simulating physical presence may not matter so long as clinical encounters maintain professional standards. But what if the distinction between doing things and merely experiencing them is important? Then, as simulations begin to efface or supersede any original, persons may depend on moral bioenhancement to enable them to stay mindful that the landscapes are simulated realities into which they risk withdrawing. Given such precautions, there is potential to enhance virtual reality systems in which users interact with computer software and expand online connectivity. For example, smartphones and telemedicine can facilitate patient access to health care and enable clinicians to return to caring for patients – including those with restricted mobility – in their own homes and communities. In the future, interactive touch technologies that digitize the sense of touch may even enable users to feel something not physically there. Together, bioenhancement and ethical use of ethical technologies hold the promise of managing new intimacies and an altered sense of reality in quasi-private spaces, where concerns also persist over personal security and privacy.

Assessment of progress

I have discussed preconditions for the operational development of person-centred health care, suggesting how values of this practice model and personal virtues and good character can be learnt and given voice. A key next step is to assess progress toward making these changes through formative and summative assessment of the internalization of core values and the possession of relevant virtues. Informal judgements of the goodness of persons take place every day, of course, but with varying degrees of success. For purposes such as educational review and health care regulation, formal tools have been developed therefore to measure character and person-centred health care practice.[58]

These assessments are complex. Current tools for measuring person-centred health care as a complete practice model, such as the Person-centred Care Assessment Tool (P-CAT),[59] tend to focus on beliefs, preferences, experiences and proxy-based outcomes of this care, often for older persons; yet people frequently cannot provide comprehensive accounts of their thinking. Moreover, the assessment tools reflect very different and rarely well-developed understandings of person-centredness, making them difficult to interpret, use and compare in health research and practice. Even measurement tools for *patient*-centred health care are evident in recent reviews of the approaches and tools available for measuring person-centred care;[58,60,61] and I am concerned that the term 'measurement' itself restricts assessment options to quantification, excluding potentially rich insights from qualitative evaluation.

Other evaluation tools focus on components of person-centred health care. For the patient–clinician relationship, they include the Person-Centred Communication Coding System,[62] and a measure of reciprocated caring between clinicians and patients.[63] Additional tools have been developed to indicate individual traits of good character, such as trust among clinicians and patients. For example, tools measuring trust by patients in their physician include the Patient Trust Scale,[64] the Patient Trust in their Physician Scale,[65] the Interpersonal Physician Trust Scale[66] and the Wake Forest Physician Trust Scale.[67] Related tools assess patient trust in physicians in particular specialties[68] and trust in people in general.[69] Using these tools in combination with a tool assessing physician trust in the patient[70] can indicate mutual trust and hence moral equality, in patient–clinician relationships.

Tending to rely on self-reports, however, such assessment tools are prone to a range of cognitive biases including self-deception and social desirability. Moral dilemmas offer an alternative way to assess the presence of virtue, but the evidence they indicate of moral reasoning ability might not equate in turn to moral action. The best evidence that clinicians and patients have of personal qualities such as trust can be expected to come from triangulating, at different times and sites, objective measurements and qualitative data gathered from sources including observations, interviews, notes and documents. In this context – and building on my work with Vikki Entwistle to develop indicators of core virtues in clinical practice[52] – Table 8.1 suggests sample indicators of the modest foundational values and virtues identified in Chapter 7, which can be assessed relationally for clinicians and patients to meet agreed priorities of these persons in their situation. Indicators of the virtues in each party have been developed to represent two directions of care in the clinician–patient relationship: self to other

Table 8.1 Sample indicators of clinician and patient virtues in the clinician–patient relationship

Values of person-centred health care	Virtues of the clinician or patient	Direction of care in the clinician–patient relationship			
		Clinician to patient	Patient to self	Clinician to self	Patient to clinician
Flourishing	Self-actualization	Recognizes the patient as a person	Achieves 'flow'	Is self-reflexive	Recognizes the clinician as a person
Personalism	Humanity	Individualizes care	Displays a good self-concept	Practises self-care activities	Respects personal boundaries
Virtue	Prudence	Takes account of the patient's life circumstances	Keeps a gratitude diary	Is self-forgiving	Is polite
Moral Equality	Justice	Treats patients as moral equals	Considers themselves equal to others	Has a personal clinician	Expresses gratitude
Pænism	Fortitude, humour	Uses humour to reduce suffering	Lives life as an adventure	Takes vacations	Smiles
Authenticity	Good faith	Communicates honestly	Minimizes unhealthy self-deception	Acts conscientiously	Discloses all relevant information
Consilience	Excellence	Exhibits humanistic skills	Is an expert patient	Balances work and life	Shows empathy

and self to self. I have reintroduced this structure from our earlier tool[63] and from Chapters 2 to 5 to contextualize variation in the influence of virtue across social roles in clinical encounters. Use of the indicators requires quantitative and qualitative assessments for research and clinical practice.

Consider, for example, assessments of moral equality through the clinician and patient trusting each other and themselves. One indicator of the component of clinician trust in patients is the extent to which the clinician trusts them to adhere to agreed treatments. Frequent follow-up assessments of patient adherence (vis-à-vis treatment effectiveness) could indicate lack of trust by the clinician. In contrast, from the perspective of the Russian proverb, 'trust but verify', at least occasional follow-up is expected of good clinicians in order to justify their level of trust. Contextualizing the appropriateness of this clinician trust is whether patients have a history of keeping appointments and setting and achieving challenging but feasible goals for their health. These indicators can be assessed objectively through medical records, and subjectively through patient self-reports, interviews and observation, for example of patients' body language (even though it can be difficult to read). Much more work is needed, however, to develop person-centred evaluation methodologies for health care. Progress here may benefit from a framework that I published for evaluating the person-centredness of different study designs.[71] This 5Cs framework suggested a need to consider using designs whose person-centredness is indicated by being case-oriented, co-constructed, caring, contextualized and complete.

Balancing

Congruence between patients' priorities and professional standards is likely when patients and clinicians share the same deep moral values.[72] Inevitably however, multifaceted and complex values and interests sometimes pull patients and clinicians in opposing directions, as exemplified by potential tension between patient autonomy, clinician beneficence and societal security. Common sense then requires balancing the rival interests to relieve moral dissonance and tension and promote mutual and interdependent welfare. Evidence of the clinician and ideally the patient developing good character facilitates their shared capability to achieve balancing. Indeed, if the colour white symbolizes virtue – as in Malcolm's claim that 'Black Macbeth will seem as pure as snow' when people compare them – then the kind of assessment described by Table 8.1 sketches a white prescription for balancing.

The table indicates virtuous behaviour that the person-centred clinician and patient commonly need to exhibit in order to share and assess or weigh opposing interests, and cooperate to construct unified preferences. Reconciliation of moral interests through balancing as a decision-making heuristic allows the strong interests of neither the clinician nor the patient to overpower countervailing interests of the other party. Unequal interests of the patient and clinician are balanced when they consensually inform a solution that satisfies each party's divergent expectations and concerns. Such a solution resolves temporary imbalance, protects the natural order of moral equality inherent to personhood, and provides stability and meaning for optimal clinician–patient interaction and mutual flourishing. The 'multi-perspective' approach of values-based health care[73-75] similarly emphasizes using social processes to facilitate balanced decision-making within clinical encounters. These processes respect the values and interests of the clinician and patient. However, my approach adds the requirement to develop virtuous persons who maximize their joint capabilities to balance competing interests by optimizing situationally just outcomes. Because these capabilities vary, the balancing tends to be asymmetrical.

In art, asymmetrical balance means that different elements of a composition offset each other, carry equal visual weight and produce a sense of harmony overall. In content, form and lighting, for example, Johannes Vermeer's painting, *Woman holding a balance*, asymmetrically balances its elements, including an empty pair of fine scales at equilibrium. Likewise, person-centred health care exemplifies asymmetrical balance. The relationship between clinicians and patients remains asymmetrical in its distribution of resources and power in favour of the clinician (despite role convergence and reduced social distances between them). However, assumed on the basis of their personhood to have equal moral interests, the clinician and patient can weigh their different interests – even if this means presenting facts on one side and opinion on the other – to make balanced treatment decisions. In the absence of intervening obstacles, these decisions can be implemented and mutually satisfying. Asymmetrical balance is evident to the extent that the clinician and patient trust, apprehend, and reconcile or stabilize moral weights for their different interests. In this close but unequal relationship, patients can trust the clinician as a confidante who will treat private and intimate details of their lives safely and effectively. Each party sees the other as another self who pulls their weight in the same direction so that the moral force of their movement enables them to flourish or at least be no worse off.

Balancing is a commonplace practice that is familiar and intuitively meaningful to persons. Clinicians and patients already negotiate and self-balance (inter) personal interests in their personal and work life. However, I envisage that asymmetrical balancing of interests in the person-centred clinician–patient relationship depends for its success on virtuous discourse as a communicative process grounded in moral values and good character. Inclusive, democratic and relational, this discourse begins with dialogue and may proceed to deliberation. Each form of open inquiry goes beyond analytic thinking to include prudential reasoning. This reasoning includes, and achieves, epistemic justification through maximizing coherence with other relevant moral virtues, as well as emotion and moral intuition.

Dialogue takes place when the clinician and patient (or agent) meet as persons who respect each other's uniqueness but also each other's moral equality. Within a relationship of mutual recognition, they work together to explore issues that require discussion. The purpose of this exploration is to bring their beliefs, values and assumptions out into the open; build joint understanding of them; and freely and safely explore differences and common ground, since interests cannot be considered until they are expressed and apprehended. Thus, the emphasis of the dialogue is on discovery and learning of values, preferences and research, not persuasion and judgement. To resolve differences and problem-solve when each party is concerned about its own and the other party's outcomes, deliberation can follow dialogue.

Deliberation can both debate the nature and significance of relevant criteria for choosing between preferences, and reconcile or integrate them with the best available research evidence. Jack Dowie and his colleagues[76] have demonstrated how, in patient-centred decision-making, online decision support can use practical and user-friendly software to implement this process to generate the best estimates available of how well each preference option performs; and this approach could extend to include clinician-specific preferences. However, limitations on the ability to quantify all preferences beg the opportunity to integrate quantitative and qualitative methods. A synthesis matrix, for example, could use numbers to tabulate the level of agreement between qualitative and quantitative evidence.

Inherent to dialogue and deliberation are the virtues developed and exercised by the clinician and patient. These virtues include these parties developing the practical wisdom to listen politely to, question respectfully, reflect fairly on, and negotiate in good faith the values and perspectives of the other person(s) alongside their own position. Such negotiation may be achieved through cooperative strategies that include trading, logrolling (or compromise when there is a moral imperative to find a solution) and, in particular, bridging – the epitome of interest-based negotiation that respects the moral equality of the patient and clinician, and related notions such as reciprocated caring.

When the positions of the clinician and patient differ significantly, *bridging* creatively crosses the decision gap between them by striving to produce a new decision option of high joint benefit. This option is an integrative moral agreement that provides the greatest good overall for both parties. In also strengthening the clinician–patient relationship, the agreement is unlikely to be repudiated once reached. Bridging requires the clinician and patient to refocus on their key common interests to reframe their positions on the most significant issues dividing them. Neither party compromises its deep values but mutual concessions on low priority matters may be required of the clinician and patient, who may also choose to 'agree to disagree' on intractable issues. Strategies to facilitate and achieve bridging vary with the type of constraint to overcome. For example, time constraints on taking preferred options can be overcome by implementing options in either an alternate or contingent sequence.[77]

In the diabetes example given at the start of the chapter, the clinician and Candy drew on their shared interest in protecting Candy's health without compromising her personhood. Consistent with the values and virtues indicated in Table 8.1, they separated this unifying interest from their different starting positions on how tightly they should aim to control her blood sugar. Then they creatively and respectfully explored ways to make healthy lifestyle changes fun and feasible for Candy, resolving her concerns about burden, loss of identity and risks to health. The example illustrates how an unmet opportunity exists to introduce bridging and other approaches to integrative negotiation into clinical practice, as well as education – for example through role-playing. These approaches can be developed and implemented as part of a larger focus on enabling students to acquire and exercise practical wisdom as an embodied process of intellectual and moral judgement, known as prudence or phronesis.

Rather than adhere to predetermined and prescriptive rules, clinicians and other persons need to learn to draw on prudence in particular, concrete circumstances. Otherwise they risk making situationally immoral decisions, even for ostensibly moral reasons. Prudence can protect against this hazard by guiding orchestration of the different virtues in order to assess and bridge moral goals and ends. Through prudence therefore, as a meta-virtue, persons exercise 'the capacity or disposition to select the right means and the right balance between means and good ends'.[78] Without prudence, those who love justice, for example, will not necessarily know, in their situation, what is just and how best to balance justice against other virtues such as courage and forgiveness. According to Aristotle, prudence is taught, guides virtuous reflection and through experience eventually becomes a habit.

Similarly, I see prudence as shaped over time by all moral learning, including integrated formal and informal curricula and recourse to moral exemplars in a nurturing moral community. Mitigating in this context the unequal distribution across clinicians and patients of material prerequisites for reasoned thinking, and the presence of uncertainty and risk, the meaning and scope of prudence go beyond practical reasoning. As conceptualized using dual process theory from cognitive and social psychology, prudence links fast, intuitive thinking, or *nous*, as tacit knowing from associative memory (System 1) and a conscious, controllable and reflective process of slow and rational thinking (System 2). Prudence further promises an Apollonian–Dionysian balance between the forces of reason and emotion, and many other virtues such as justice and good faith.[79] This inclusive conception of prudence accommodates for clinicians and patients a role for both conscious and intuitive unconscious judgements to inform intentions and future action.[80] Although prone to producing biased or inaccurate and unverifiable judgements,[81] intuitions can be personally meaningful and significant, and acquire credibility, under certain conditions. These conditions include lived experience and the absence of strong research evidence, especially of complex, ill-defined and time-limited situations. Values, virtues and reasons here may not be fully and easily articulated but may be made mutually understandable by imagining oneself in the position of the other person. Based on processes of direct and indirect perception, intuition then may insightfully and universally mediate the use of reason and emotions as appraisal mechanisms, in particular, individual cases of communication. In this context, persons may also learn to recognize when System 1 thinking risks leading deliberations astray, requiring System 2 thinking that is slow, analytic and effortful. New situations with which the person is unfamiliar, or tension between virtues, may also require

System 2 thinking. For example, a patient might want to offer a gift to his clinician out of gratitude, but be uncertain the first time whether or how to do so out of fear the clinician will question the motivation for, and appropriateness of, the gift-giving.

Conclusion

Implementing person-centred health care requires producing social conditions conducive to clinicians and patients developing and exercising virtues and good character. These conditions include social structures and processes within families, schools and the community as well as new and emergent technologies. Virtue is conceived here less as a skill to be learnt in the classroom than as a way of being and everyday living into which persons can be socialized and enculturated at all levels of society. Assessment of progress toward meeting these goals will require developing and integrating evaluation tools and related approaches – quantitative and qualitative – for use in health care practice and research. Evaluation then can indicate good character among clinicians and patients, who are relationally disposed in their circumstances to practise the virtues and live good lives together. Nevertheless, how virtue can best balance the welfare of the clinician and patient will now demand empirical attention.

References

1 Arthur J, Kristjánsson K, Thomas H, Kotzee B, Ignatowicz A, Qiu T. Virtuous medical practice. Birmingham Jubilee Centre for Character and Virtues, University of Birmingham 2015.
2 McKalip D. Pay for performance and public reporting: risks to patients outweigh benefits. *Journal of American Physicians and Surgeons* 2009; 14: 113–7.
3 Sandel M. Liberalism and republicanism: friends or foes? A reply to Richard Dagger. *The Review of Politics* 1999; 61: 209–14.
4 Donetto S, Pierri P, Tsianakas V, Roberts G. Experience-based co-design and health-care improvement: realizing participatory design in the public sector. *Design Journal* 2015; 18: 227–48.
5 Smith C. *To Flourish or Destruct.* Chicago: University of Chicago Press; 2015.
6 Narvaez D. The co-construction of virtue. In: Snow N, editor. *Cultivating Virtue: Perspectives from Philosophy, Theology, and Psychology.* New York: Oxford University Press; 2014. pp. 251–78.
7 Govrin A. From ethics of care to psychology of care: reconnecting ethics of care to contemporary moral psychology. *Frontiers in Psychology* 2014; 5.
8 Thompson R. The development of virtue. In: Snow N, editor. *Cultivating Virtue: Perspectives from Philosophy, Theology, and Psychology.* New York: Oxford University Press; 2014. pp. 279–306.
9 Hilton S. *More Human. Designing a World Where People Come First.* London: WH Allen; 2015.
10 Cohen J. Social, emotional, ethical and academic education: creating a climate for learning, participation in democracy, and well-being. *Harvard Educational Review* 2006; 76: 201–37.

11 Arthur J. *Of Good Character: Exploration of Virtues and Values in 3–25 Year-Olds*. Exeter: Imprint Academic; 2003.

12 Arthur J, Kristjánsson K, Walker D, Sanderse W, Jones C. Character Education in UK Schools. Birmingham Jubilee Centre for Character and Virtue, University of Birmingham 2015.

13 Leininger M. *Cultural Care Diversity and Universality. A Theory of Nursing*. New York: National League for Nursing Press; 1991.

14 Watson J. Watson's philosophy and theory of human caring in nursing. In: Riehl-Sisca J, editor. *Conceptual Models for Nursing Practice*. Third edition. Norwalk: Appleton and Lange; 1989. pp. 219–36.

15 Boykin A, Schoenhofer S. *Nursing as Caring: A Model for Transforming Practice*. New York: National League for Nursing Press.

16 Roach S. *Caring: The Human Mode of Being*. Toronto: University of Toronto; 1984.

17 McCormack B, McCance T. *Person-Centred Nursing: Theory and Practice*. Oxford: Wiley-Blackwell; 2010.

18 Kitwood T. *Dementia Reconsidered: The Person comes First*. Buckingham: Open University Press; 1997.

19 McWhinney I. *A Textbook of Family Medicine*. Oxford: Oxford University Press; 1997.

20 Taylor M. *Hippocrates Cried: The Decline of American Psychiatry*. Oxford: Oxford University Press.

21 Janssen A, MacLeod R. Who cares for whom? Reciprocity of care at the end of life. *Journal of Palliative Care and Medicine* 2012; 2: 129; doi:10.4172/2165-7386. 1000129.

22 Horton R. A new epoch for health professionals' education. *Lancet* 2010; 376: 1875–7.

23 Mezzich J, Đorđević V, Braš M, Appleyard J. The Zagreb Congress and whole person health education and training. *International Journal of Person Centered Medicine* 2014; 4: 1–5.

24 Horton R. *Second Opinion*. London: Granta Books; 2003.

25 Buetow S. The virtue of uncertainty in health care. *Journal of Evaluation in Clinical Practice* 2011; 17: 873–6.

26 Gupta M, Upshur R. Critical thinking in clinical medicine: what is it? *Journal of Evaluation in Clinical Practice* 2012; 18: 938–44.

27 Coulehan J. You say self-interest, I say altruism. In: Wear D, Aultman JM, editors. *Professionalism in Medicine: Critical Perspectives*. New York: Springer; 2006. pp. 103–27.

28 Wilkinson T, Wade W. A blueprint to assess professionalism: results of a systematic review. *Academic Medicine* 2009; 84: 551–8.

29 Carey G, Curlin F, Yoon J. Medical student opinions on character development in medical education: a national survey. *BMC Research Notes* 2015; 8: 455–60.

30 Shapiro J. Does medical education promote professional alexithymia? A call for attending to the emotions of patients and self in medical training. *Academic Medicine* 2011; 86: 326–32.

31 Branch W. Supporting the moral development of medical students. *Journal of General Internal Medicine* 2000; 15: 503–8.

32 Kristjánsson K. Ten myths about character, virtue and virtue education – plus three well-founded misgivings. *British Journal of Educational Studies* 2013; 61: 269–87.

33 Cottingham A, Suchman A, Litzelman D, Frankel R, Mossbarger D, Williamson P, Baldwin D, Inui T. Enhancing the informal curriculum of a medical school: a case

study in organizational culture change. *Journal of General Internal Medicine* 2008; 23: 715–22.

34 Branch W, Kern D, Haidet P, Weissmann P, Gracey C, Mitchell G, Inui T. Teaching the human dimensions of care in clinical settings. *Journal of the American Medical Association* 2001; 286: 1067–74.

35 Charon R. Narrative medicine: a model for empathy, reflection, profession, and trust. *Journal of the American Medical Association* 2001; 286: 1897–902.

36 Novack D, Suchman A, Clark W, Epstein R, Najberg E, Kaplan C. Calibrating the physician: personal awareness and effective patient care. *Journal of the American Medical Association* 1997; 278: 502–9.

37 Litzelman DK, Cottingham AH. The new formal competency-based curriculum and informal curricula at Indiana University School of Medicine: overview and five-year analysis. *Academic Medicine* 2007; 82: 410–21.

38 Lown BA, Manning CF. The Schwartz Center Rounds: evaluation of an interdisciplinary approach to enhancing patient-centered communication, teamwork, and provider support. *Academic Medicine* 2010; 85: 1073–81.

39 Blumenfeld B. Engaging Students with Havruta Style Learning. *Institute for Law Teaching and Learning*. 2011; Available at: http://lawteaching.org/conferences/2011/ handouts/2b- EngagingStudentswithHavruta.pdf. Accessed 21 March 2015.

40 Jacob J. Exercise and gardening programs as tools to reduce community violence. *Journal of the American Medical Association* 2015; 314: 1435–7.

41 Aristotle. *The Nicomachean Ethics.* Fifth edition. London: Kegan Paul; 1893.

42 Boler M. *Feeling power: Emotions and education.* New York: Routledge; 1999.

43 Wear D. Respect for patients. In: Wear D, Aultman J, editors. *Professionalism in Medicine.* New York: Springer; 2006. pp. 87–101.

44 Frank A. Reflective healthcare practice. In: Kinsella EA, Pitman A, editors. *Phronesis as Professional Knowledge.* Rotterdam: Sense Publishers; 2012. pp. 53–60.

45 Rest JR. *Development in Judging Moral issues.* Minneapolis: University of Minnesota Press; 1979.

46 Haidt J. Moral psychology for the twenty-first century. *Journal of Moral Education* 2013; 42: 281–97.

47 Sulmasy D. What is conscience and why is respect for it so important? *Theoretical Medicine and Bioethics* 2008; 29: 135–49.

48 Ekman I, Hedman H, Swedberg K, Wallengren C. Commentary: Swedish initiative on person centred care. *British Medical Journal* 2015; 350: h160.

49 Tonelli MR. Person-centered care in intensive care medicine. *International Journal of Person Centered Medicine* 2013; 3: 23–6.

50 Slote M. The roots of empathy. In: Snow N, editor. *Cultivating virtue: Perspectives from Philosophy, Theology, and Psychology.* Oxford: Oxford University Press; 2014. pp. 65–84.

51 Buetow S, Elwyn G. Patient performance standards: the next bold policy initiative in health care? *Journal of Health Services Research and Policy* 2007; 12: 48–53.

52 Buetow S, Entwistle V. Pay-for-virtue: an option to improve pay-for-performance? *Journal of Evaluation in Clinical Practice* 2011; 17: 894–8.

53 Charlton BG. Genospirituality: genetic engineering for spiritual and religious enhancement. *Medical Hypotheses* 2008; 71: 825–8.

54 Walker M. Enhancing genetic virtue: a project for twenty-first century humanity? *Politics and the Life Sciences* 2009; 28: 27–47.

55 Specker J, Focquaert F, Raus K, Sterckx S, Schermer M. The ethical desirability of moral bioenhancement: a review of reasons. *BMC Medical Ethics* 2014; 15.

56 Nayar P. *Posthumanism.* Cambridge, UK: Polity Press; 2014.

57 Agar N. *Truly Human Enhancement: A Philosophical Defense of Limits.* Cambridge, MA: MIT Press; 2014.

58 de Silva, D for The Health Foundation. Helping measure person-centred care. Evidence review. London: The Evidence Centre; 2014.

59 Edvardsson D, Fetherstonhaugh D, Nay R, Gibson S. Development and initial testing of the Person-centred Care Assessment Tool (P-CAT). *International Psychogeriatrics* 2010; 22: 101–8.

60 Leyns C, De Maeseneer J. Conceptualizing person- and people-centeredness in primary health care: a literature review. *International Journal of Person Centered Medicine* 2013; 3: 13–22.

61 National Quality Forum. Priority setting for healthcare performance measurement: addressing performance measure gaps in person-centered care and outcomes. Final report. Washington DC: National Quality Forum; 2014.

62 Ledoux T, Hilmers A, Watson K, Baranowski T, O'Connor TM. Development and feasibility of an objective measure of patient-centered communication fidelity in a pediatric obesity intervention. *Journal of Nutrition Education and Behaviour* 2013; 45: 349–54.

63 Buetow S, Fuehrer A, Macfarlane K, McConnell D, Moir F, Huggard P, Doerr H. Development and validation of a patient measure of doctor–patient caring. *Patient Education and Counseling* 2012; 86: 264–9.

64 Kao AC, Green DC, Zaslavsky AM, Koplan JP, Cleary PD. The relationship between method of physician payment and patient trust. *Journal of the American Medical Association* 1998; 280: 1708–14.

65 Leisen B, Hyman MR. An improved scale for assessing patients' trust in their physician. *Health Marketing Quarterly* 2001; 19: 23–42.

66 Hall MA, Dugan E, Zheng B, Mishra AK. Trust in physicians and medical institutions: what is it, can it be measured, and does it matter? *Milbank Quarterly* 2001; 79: 613–39.

67 Hall MA, Zheng B, Dugan E, Camacho F, Kidd KE, Mishra A, Balkrishnan R. Measuring patients' trust in their primary care providers. *Medical Care Research and Review* 2002; 59: 293–318.

68 Hillen MA, Butow PN, Tattersall MH, Hruby G, Boyle FM, Vardy J, Kallimanis-King BL, de Haes HC, Smets EM. Validation of the English version of the Trust in Oncologist Scale (TiOS). *Patient Education and Counseling* 2013; 91: 25–8.

69 Yamagishi T, Yamagishi M. Trust and commitment in the United States and Japan. *Motivation and Emotion* 1994; 18: 129–66.

70 Thom D, Wong S, Guzman D, Wu A, Penko A, Miaskowski C, Kushel, M. Physician trust in the patient: Development and validation of a new measure. *Annals of Family Medicine* 2011; 9: 148–54.

71 Buetow S. A framework for doing person-centred health research. *International Journal of Person Centered Medicine* 2011; 1: 358–61.

72 Veatch R. Abandoning informed consent. *Hastings Center Report* 1995; 25: 5–12.

73 Little M, Gordon J, Lipworth W, Markham P, Kerridge I. Values as 'modest foundations' for medicine. *European Journal for Person Centered Healthcare* 2014; 2: 154–61.

74 Fulford KWM. Ten principles of value-based medicine. In: Schramme T, Thome J, editors. *Philosophy and Psychiatry.* Berlin: Die Deutsche Bibliothek; 2004. pp. 50–80.

75 Fulford KWM. Values-based practice: Fulford's dangerous idea. *Journal of Evaluation in Clinical Practice* 2013; 19: 537–46.

76 Dowie J, Kaltoft MK, Salkeld G, Cunich M. Towards generic online multicriteria decision support in patient centred health care. *Health Expectations* 2013; 18: 689–702.

77 Buetow S. Four strategies for negotiated care. *Journal of the Royal Society of Medicine* 1998; 91: 199–201.

78 Pellegrino ED, Thomasma DC. *The Virtues in Medical Practice.* New York: Oxford University Press; 1993.

79 Braude H. *Intuition in Medicine. A Philosophical Defense of Clinical Reasoning.* Chicago: University of Chicago Press; 2012.

80 Buetow S, Mintoft B. When should patient intuition be taken seriously? *Journal of General Internal Medicine* 2011; 26: 433–6.

81 Redelmeier DA, Schull MJ, Hux JE, Tu JV, Ferris LE. Problems for clinical judgment: 1. Eliciting an insightful history of present illness. *Canadian Medical Association Journal* 2001; 164: 647–51.

Index